Insight and Love

Insight and Love

An introduction to Insight meditation—a practical way to become free from emotional conflict

with selected essays

Graham Williams, Ph.D.

Lifeflow® Publications

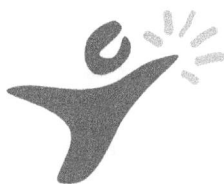

the **Life**flow
meditation centre

First published in Australia 1988 by Kurlana Publishing
Reprinted in 1994

This revised edition 2007 published by
Lifeflow® Publications
Unit 8 / 259 Glen Osmond Rd
Frewville SA 5063
Australia

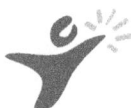

the **Life**flow
meditation centre

ISBN:978-0-9804562-0-2.
Printed in Australia.
Cover and book design by Steven Parashis of Designad
Cover image: original ink brush artwork *Joy* by John Burston

Print book and ebook distributed by DoctorZed Publishing
www.doctorzed.com

This book is dedicated with undying gratitude for their enormous generosity, to the memory of my teachers in the Kargyu lineage:

His Holiness the 16th Karmapa
Kalu Rinpoche
Namgyal Rinpoche
Chorpel and Sonam

Acknowledgements

I thank Louise Niva for all her help and support in bringing this book to life many years ago.
I also thank and am very grateful to Gretta Koch for bringing her editing skills to cleaning up my text for this edition and John Burston for reading it through.

CONTENTS

Introduction   **I**

Chapter 1   Raising the question
                INTERLUDE 1: *The body as a teacher*   **1**

Chapter 2   Why meditation?
                INTERLUDE 2: *The gift of solitude*   **17**

Chapter 3   Preparation—simplifying the life
                INTERLUDE 3: *Work is the sign of friendship*   **33**

Chapter 4   Foundation—sustaining the question
                INTERLUDE 4: *The question of love*   **55**

Chapter 5   Calm and concentration—balancing body
                and mind   **87**

Chapter 6   Meditations for developing calm
                and concentration   **98**

Chapter 7   Clear and open—beyond answers
                Meditations for developing insight
                INTERLUDE 5: *The story of the diamond*   **111**

Chapter 8   Integration, a life of love—going beyond
                wanting and fear
                INTERLUDE 6: *Kindness and gentleness*   **129**

For the first time you see reality without thinking about it and without any self-referencing whatsoever. Experiencing this for the first time is quite a shock; it's a revelation which is exhilarating, incredibly simple, a great relief and even hilariously funny.

I wrote this book in 1986 during a year's retreat at The Lifeflow Meditation Centre's mallee sanctuary in the Riverland in South Australia. Because of this, the writing is very concentrated, direct and, as a friend of mine commented, "There's no 'I' in it". I was focused on Insight meditation at the time, so my writing tends to be rather pithy.

Insight meditation produces a state where you see clearly and directly by stripping away everything else. It's a process of removing all the layers until the core of your mind is revealed—crystalline and clear. Insight is cool rather than warm. It's for seeing. And this book reflects that state.

However, I decided not to change the text. I've always felt that any piece of work, whether music, writing or painting, has its integrity at the time it is created, and to attempt to change it later can destroy that. The book is composed so that each chapter is followed by an interlude. The essays that make up the interludes were written during the same year, and therefore reflect on the same themes, ideas and experiences outlined in the main text.

These short essays can be read separately, or as a commentary on the main text, or can be passed over altogether if you wish. They make the distinction between love and security and follow the theme of letting go; of opening up and consciously learning to be receptive. Their focus is on learning to *be* instead of always having to *do*—going "inwards and downwards" instead of "onwards and upwards".

In the West we all learn how to get things together in our lives—how to build things up, how to succeed and grow, and hold on to what we have. I like to sum up our cultural tradition as "onwards and upwards". We are very good at it. But we don't see that life doesn't always work this way—it's only half the story. As every move we make eventually balances itself, everything that goes up must come down. So the other half of the story is "inwards and downwards".

We believe that what we have built, whether physically or in a career or in a relationship, must not change, must not come unstuck—we have to hold it all together. But of course everything does change and come unstuck. The meditation tradition provides a way to come unstuck skilfully, gracefully and enjoyably. You can learn to go inwards and downwards just as masterfully as you learned to go onwards and upwards.

When you experience this, it dawns on you that being stuck is actually a very painful position to be in. Becoming unstuck, when you learn not to be afraid of it, is extremely blissful. It provides enormous relief, as you discover that the feeling of going in and down accompanies the process of the mind and body regaining their natural balance. Your energies are restored and refreshed. You are completely open to the rich world of your senses and have access to the infinite detail and variety they reveal, which you normally do not notice, and to the world of your intuition.

*   *   *

Although I trained for ten years in the Buddhist meditation traditions of Burma and Tibet, I was not at all attracted to the cultural and religious beliefs or structures of Buddhism but to the practical knowledge and experience which form the discipline of these traditions. Therefore everything I have taught and written, including this book, is completely free from the inherent jargon which tends to come with anything Buddhist.

This book is based on the practical teaching of Buddhism, which is a discipline to understand the cause of the underlying conflicting emotions that drive human life, and become free from them. I became interested in this discipline because I achieved everything I dreamed of and found it did not make the slightest difference to how I felt internally. I also noticed that neither greatness and brilliance nor a happy marriage guaranteed wisdom or emotional maturity. In fact, often greatness and fame increased insecurity.

It was written at the request of my teacher, Namgyal Rinpoche, after he led a retreat based on the book *The Mahamudra, Eliminating the darkness of ignorance* (Library of Tibetan Works and Archives, Dharamsala, 1978, translated by Alexander Berzin) by the ninth Karmapa (Wangchug Dorje). The Karmapa is the head of the Karma Kargyu lineage of Tibetan Buddhism and the title passes from generation to generation—the ninth Karmapa lived in the sixteenth century. I found this text straightforward and practical, accepting the cultural differences, so have used it as a reference ever since, particularly when testing and explaining the experiences and realisations of students in Insight meditation.

Mahamudra means literally, "great movement" and also "great seal". It is a system of study and practice designed to bring about the direct experience of the fundamental, infinite and clear state of our natural consciousness. This experience is called "emptiness" or "openness" and is the core realisation of all Buddhist practice and the "great seal" of Mahamudra. It is the direct experience and seeing of your own mind when it is completely still and free from thoughts—so it is "empty" of concepts or completely "open". From here you perceive the world in the same way, without any thought or self-referencing, and so "empty" of concepts or again, "open" or transparent.

The openness and clarity of consciousness is experienced in four distinct "seals" or stages. This is the core practice of Insight meditation and I explain it in chapter 7. I also describe all the preparatory practices for experiencing the four stages of insight outlined in the Mahamudra tradition. These are explained in a very brief and concentrated form to make them easier to understand and therefore more accessible.

The practice of Tantra is used to integrate the living experience of these four stages by realising a fifth "seal" of the natural radiance of consciousness—its vibrant, luminous quality. Experiencing for yourself the four different stages of insight into the nature of consciousness, and integrating the fifth level of its radiant state, is the aim of Insight meditation and Tantra. Insight and Tantra complement each other. With Insight you see through the hopes and fears which have always bedevilled human life. With Tantra you embrace life fully and use Insight to ride and transform the emotions that drive us.

*   *   *

Into the fabric of the text are woven the ideas of Western philosophy and psychology, particularly those of the philosophers Bertrand Russell and Jean-Paul Sartre, and the Swiss psychologist Carl Jung. I have linked Insight meditation with our own philosophic tradition, because it is based on the same foundation of question—of not taking anything for granted.

However, what I found unique about Buddhism was its practical meditation tradition where you learn skills in order to gain direct knowledge and experience of how our minds and emotions actually work. You have a teacher with whom everything can be tested, so there is no question of having to believe anything. You have either experienced something or you haven't, and it can be tested, repeated and sustained.

Here is a system of knowledge and practical techniques for discovering how human consciousness actually works. The difference from any Western form of psychological knowledge is that you actually study your own mind and can experience for yourself direct insight into the way consciousness works and how your perceptions operate. It is a method and form of knowledge unique to the East, and I have come to the conviction that it can be fruitfully integrated into our own culture.

Buddhism also has a rich tradition of psychology and philosophy. Many of the psychological concepts of Buddhism are now being incorporated into modern psychology, and more people have become familiar with the philosophical concepts because of the discoveries in quantum physics. However, what makes the meditation tradition so different from anything in our own culture is the fact that this knowledge is not gained by studying the world, human beings and the mind as objects. It comes from actually experiencing yourself.

You can discover how thinking actually works; see the mind when it is still and has no thoughts in it; see the relationship between your mind and body and between your mind and the objects you are looking at, and see what concepts are and how they affect the perceptions you have of the world. Unlike our own tradition where these things are studied as ideas, here they are tangible experiences that you can feel, see and experience in your own body, here and now.

None of this knowledge is theoretic, because it is based on the very simple premise that it is impossible to know the human mind only by studying others objectively. We are it. The only way to understand human emotions, mental processes and consciousness itself is to have some way of observing our own. And this is what meditation, and the techniques of Insight meditation in particular, enable you to do.

This process can then be extended because it is possible to add to our objective knowledge of the world by understanding that we are an integral part of that as well. The methods and techniques of the meditation tradition can add the missing subjective observations.

Being able to directly experience these things has a profound effect on your life. No longer are these theories, ideas and possibilities just questions which remain divorced from your actual experience. They become embodied, literally, as you feel them and make the connections in yourself between emotions, thoughts, feelings, sensations and concepts. Instead of living only in the mind, working with the ideas of philosophy or having to believe the dogmas of religion, you discover that your *whole body* is conscious.

Your life changes from feeling busy mentally, and either feeling nothing at all or just empty in the body, to being able to experience both your body and mind as completely integrated. You then know, and can sustain as a living, direct and ever-present experience what the meditation tradition means by "radiant presence".

This totally overhauls our Western ideas of consciousness and, in fact, philosophers are just starting to question our notions of consciousness in these terms. You discover that it is something fundamental to life, and to your life in particular. This is what is meant by "the great seal" mentioned earlier. It is the direct experience of consciousness as the foundation of all your physical and mental processes.

*   *   *

This book also covers in summary the different streams of the Buddhist meditation tradition. There are four of them: Calm and Concentration, Insight meditation, Tantra and Ethics. I will write in detail on each of these streams in four later books. (The first of these, outlining the stream of Calm and Concentration, is due to be completed in 2008.)

The stream of Calm and Concentration outlines all the different ways of meditating and describes the different levels of experience you can have. It's where you learn to relax your body skilfully and immediately while keeping your mind clear and alert. It begins with how and where you set yourself up to meditate, and ends with the deepest levels of meditative absorption.

Insight meditation provides the tool to concentrate the mind so that you can observe your own body, feelings, states of mind and the thoughts and processes of your mind. You can do this not only as a detached observer but also as a direct participant, from within. The goal of Insight meditation is to see, or in the case of insight itself, to *directly experience* your own mind and the world around you. What this means is that you are in a state where you can perceive things without the normal concepts, ideas, stories, hopes and fears which colour and shape your experience of yourself and life.

This is a unique state, because your mind has to be completely still, clear and balanced for this to occur. In the Insight meditation literature it's called "seeing reality as it is" or "seeing things as they really are". It might sound a bit naïve, perhaps even mundane, but I can assure you it isn't. Experiencing this for the first time is quite a shock; it's a revelation which is exhilarating, ecstatic, incredibly simple, a great relief and even hilariously funny. For the first time you see reality without thinking about it and without any self-referencing whatsoever.

The stream of Tantra is concerned with integrating insight with the living experience of your body, and outlines techniques to sustain the realisations you gain in formal meditation in every kind of situation in life. It links everything back to the body, and so brings in warmth, bliss and vitality and provides tools for maintaining a rich feeling-life. I have included the preparatory exercises from the Tibetan tantric tradition in chapter 4 as they are an integral part of Mahamudra. However, I have considerably simplified them and explained their purpose. They are not necessary for doing Insight meditation, but they can be useful for making insight a living, ongoing experience in your life.

Ethics, the fourth stream, deals with how to live happily and usefully by keeping your mind in a healthy state. Ethics in this context are not a set of arcane rules, or even intellectual propositions, but practical guidelines derived from direct insight into how our minds work. They are designed to provide support for your meditation practice and help integrate the relaxed, alert state of meditation with your everyday life.

The final chapter on integration summarises the function of Tantra. It doesn't go into any of the traditional exercises as they are not usually included in Mahamudra—I will detail these in a later book. (For example, there are visualisations, mantras and six tantric yogas, the Six Yogas of Naropa, which form an extremely interesting body of meditation practice.) The quality of mind I describe in this final chapter is the foundation of consciousness or the state of pure awareness. It is clear, open, infinite and luminous; free from concepts, thoughts and images. It is known in Tantra as *clear light*. This luminous quality of mind can be sustained beyond formal meditation practice and so enables the experience of insight—the realisation of openness—to be integrated into everyday life.

The knowledge and skill of meditation practice and the traditions of Insight meditation and Tantra were not, up until the last century, known by or available to our culture. These rich traditions are unique to the East and I feel it is important to respect and value them by realising that the East has developed the understanding of human emotions and the mind to the same extent that the West has developed science and technology.

I also think it is crucially important to see that they balance and complement the developments of the West. I have found it is possible to maintain the integrity of these practices and traditions while simplifying and adapting them to our own culture so they are easily understandable and accessible.

This book, then, is a concentrated, simple summary of the Mahamudra tradition, focusing particularly on Insight meditation. However, my aim is to integrate the tradition with our own so that, rather than something still exotic, it becomes something we can experience in our own minds and bodies, here and now.

Graham Williams
Kurlana Mallee Sanctuary
January, 2006

| *Raising the question*

It is quite possible, because of the image we have of ourselves and of the ideas surrounding meditation, not to recognise the teaching and teacher which are right in front of us. For this reason it is important to be honest about the body—where our bodies are is where we are, and nowhere else. And that is the best place to begin.

Raising the question of meditation inevitably involves raising a host of associated questions: Which method? What tradition? Which teaching? Which teacher? Where do we begin? Where does it all end? This is inevitable because the essential nature of Insight meditation is question itself. The ways and methods of meditating have thus proliferated, according to culture and temperament.

In a sense, the question of Insight meditation begins where all other questions leave off; where all questions which have an answer become dissatisfying, and when we are ready and willing to plumb the whole nature of question itself. This entails giving up the certainties and comforting half-truths with which we insulate our lives, and being prepared to face uncertainty and doubt. It means facing the constant shadow, the despair which pervades life behind the facades of distraction and respectable busyness.

Undertaking Insight meditation will therefore come from a sense of necessity, of finding intolerable the half-life dream in which life is usually played out, the waste which this involves, and the conflict and confusion which inevitably go hand in hand with ignoring the doubt associated with every certainty.

Insight meditation is the process of letting go of what we think we know, and of questioning what appears to be obvious—what we completely take for granted. It is the way of unknowing, of being prepared to question everything without restriction. It is not dependent on any creed, dogma, tradition, belief or concept, but on direct observation: the investigation of all the physical, emotional and mental aspects of our own lives.

We need to turn and face what appears to be obvious, for the obvious is the one thing which is usually ignored. Perhaps what actually *is*, is not seen clearly because it is always there, obscured by what we feel we ought to think, see or do, or by what we think we ought to feel. Perhaps the first obvious thing to face is the reality of our own death.

Insight meditation is the work of addressing ourselves to this fundamental level of questioning. This means giving up convictions, opinions and points of view because to cling to these, although they may be partially true, is to be committed to proving and defending them. Having to prove or defend anything generates conflict, both for ourselves and others. The root of this conflict lies in the fact that nothing lasts anyway, no matter how convincing our proof or valiant our defence.

*   *   *

The process of questioning involves relinquishing all fixed ideas and preconceptions. Naturally this is a very disorienting experience, and it is for this reason that the question of meditation can only come from a feeling of necessity. If we are absolutely certain of our beliefs then this question will never arise.

The first step towards questioning is an act of complete humility. We need to face the fact that in spite of all the answers and certainties the human race has erected in the name of religion, science and civilization, we are still haunted by doubt and frustration. Every answer breeds question, and every conviction is littered with the debris of dissension.

To query existence raises one of the most fundamental questions which can be asked. This brings us face to face with the body. It is an extraordinarily intricate organism about which an enormous range of facts has been collated, but which still remains a question simply by the sheer fact of its existence.

Inordinate amounts of time, effort and money are devoted to providing it with an unending supply of other life-forms through which it bites, chews and swallows its way. An equally inordinate amount of time, effort and money is dedicated to disguising the fact that these are then excreted in a degraded form and disposed of.

Why does it behave in this way? Why does our culture glorify, exaggerate and advertise one end of the process and try to hide the other with discretion, disinfectants and deodorisers? Why is one orifice so acceptable and the other not?

This raises the whole question of aesthetics and social conventions; of what is considered to be beautiful and what is ugly; of what is good and what is bad. By ranging across different cultures and periods of history it becomes clear that no universal opinion is held. Beauty and ugliness, goodness and badness, prove to be just as ephemeral and ambiguous as all other opinions.

What is beautiful at one time, particularly regarding the body, is not at another, and what one culture considers perfectly good behaviour, another considers highly improper. Entire attitudes to the body change from one period of history to another, even within the same civilisation. In our own, views of the body have ranged from seeing it as a divine image, to a machine, and then as an aggregate of animal instincts, all in the brief period of five hundred years.

*   *   *

The problem of identity arises at this point. Are we our bodies, or is there some substance contained within them which is the real "us"—a self, soul or psyche? Or are we none of these, or all of them? Do we exist at all? Could we then, with certainty, come to the conclusion that to be certain of anything is impossible?

Even this will eventually founder in the face of physical experiences like hunger and death. Perhaps life is an experience which has nothing to do with questions and answers. If this were so, then to spend our time looking for or maintaining an answer would be an appalling waste of time.

This again brings us face to face with our bodies, now seen from a completely new perspective. Instead of trying to find answers and explanations for the body's existence, the possibility of observing it, in itself, as something not final but as an ongoing process, arises. Wouldn't this open up an entirely different world? If this is true, then why doesn't everyone do it? Perhaps it is not as easy as it sounds, which could explain why acceptance of concepts and convictions is the norm.

It requires being prepared to begin again, like a child, and to see without any attempt at labelling or conceptualising. This means perceiving directly, exactly as a child does, before she or he learns language and a way of naming things. The difference between a child and an adult is that a child is unaware of the fact that this is what she or he is doing. An adult, having learned to conceptualise, has the option of returning to and re-incorporating the ability to perceive directly and nakedly, with full awareness of what is being done.

One of the major problems obstructing this direct seeing is the way in which we are educated about life—the answers were all given to us long before we got around to asking the questions. A distinction needs to be drawn between the emotional "security" invested in those answers and the process of conceptualisation itself. The invested emotions are the greatest hindrance to seeing this process clearly.

*   *   *

Perceiving directly means being totally open to sensations and feelings without any mental constructions whatsoever; registering them and allowing them to be revealed so that they might be distinguished fully and clearly. What hinders this process is our identifying with the patterns laid down by our parental and cultural conditioning (our name, family, school, city, country and so on), and as a result we cannot afford to have these patterns and constructions questioned.

So our perceptions are socially predetermined. As soon as something is named, we stop looking—it is "known". Then things can only be seen or heard in a certain way; their shapes and uses have been predetermined, and more often than not, they are only perceived in terms of how they either support or threaten the images or constructions which are laid down in the consciousness. Wanting and fear distort and actually block the process of perception, because our identity is locked into and tied up with these images.

It is impossible to perceive clearly as long as these mental constructions are ignored and held onto. We need to be prepared to let go of them, to give up identifying with them. As long as "I am" exists—I am doctor, teacher, builder, therapist, lover, businessperson, parent, child, and so on—clear seeing is totally impossible, for these images determine all of our perceptions. This creates a state of conflict between the mental image of what we think we are perceiving and what actually is.

The reason for this is that we become falsely confident by believing our labels, and so completely ignore phenomena. Ignoring the world around us is at the root of all emotional conflict, because the price of conceptualisation is believing that phenomena are fixed and actually exist separately from our mental images of them.

Believing that things exist either outside or inside ourselves, and that lasting satisfaction can be drawn from them, is the cause of emotional conflict. We believe our "knowledge" and are left wanting.

*　　*　　*

Reintegrating the ability to perceive clearly and directly necessitates a state which is totally open, attentive and observant. In this state, the need to label is relinquished. This requires the development of a deep calm and a concentration which is completely absorbed. These constitute the essence of all meditation teachings. The methods and schools proliferate in accordance with how these states are attained.

At this point we are dealing with the forces which have

shaped our thinking. The preconceptions and fixed ideas that we have inherited hinder the attaining of direct perception. It is therefore going to be difficult to recognise preconceptions if we involve ourselves in an entire reconditioning process by unquestioningly taking on a tradition from another culture when we attempt to meditate. The problem is then compounded, because another layer of conditioning has been added to the ones already there. It does not solve the problem of labelling and identification if we assume a whole new set of predetermined labels and take on another identity.

Therefore when raising the question of where to begin with meditation, it is important to look to the body. We need to let go of all the fixed ideas we might have about meditating—what we have read in books, or heard from others—and face our bodies for what they really are.

Without the body, meditation is impossible. Physically, we have been conditioned both geographically and culturally. There are certain bodily limitations. The body can only be in one place at a time. To be in a particular place while dreaming of being in another and thinking that we would be able to meditate if we were there, or only after meeting a particular teacher or master, is impossible to realise in actuality and comes to nothing but absurdity.

Observing the body without fixed ideas brings us to a point of direct honesty. If we simply dream of meditating, then we are not doing it and so the realisation of the necessity to do so has obviously not arisen. It would then be much better to do something else. If we consider it necessary to find a teacher and do not do so, then we are being evasive and are simply avoiding seeing what we are really doing. If we are content to read books and talk about meditation, then that is what we are doing and so we are still in the realm of conceptualisation divorced from experience.

It is only through facing the body that we can sort out all the questions that are raised along with meditation. An old saying states that when the student is ready, the teacher is there. In one sense this is simply pointing out the fact that when the necessity of meditating becomes apparent in our lives, the way to do so will become apparent as well.

It is quite possible, because of the image we have of ourselves and of the ideas surrounding meditation, not to recognise the teaching and teacher which are right in front of us. For this reason it is important to be honest about the body—where our bodies are is where we are, and nowhere else. And that is the best place to begin.

The stiller and quieter, the truer.

| *The body as a teacher*

Opening to the very fine sensations and feelings of our bodies is essential for a state of living calm and well-being to arise. To cut off these feelings is to be divorced from life, and to have no contact with reality.

The body is the touchstone. Here is the test-point for all insight. It is only through the body that things can be real; therefore, until something can be seen and tested in the body, it is not realised.

Our contact with life is our own body; an organism of infinite sensing capacity, which we experience through the entire skin, the tongue, nose, ears, eyes, and the mind. The basis of meditation is untying the knots which have been tied in how we perceive the experience of our senses—the knots laid down by conditioning, both personal and cultural. This is done by learning not to interfere: to open to the body, without distraction, and to listen.

Of course, when we start to open and listen, sometimes there is pain. Knots and distortions are painful. However, it is better to feel pain than to render ourselves feelingless and empty, because then the way is open and we know what we are dealing with. Not vague ideas and intuitions, but something direct.

And here is a teacher, a guide. For if we are prepared to

listen and to feel, the pain will go. Both pleasure and pain are totally interdependent—one cannot be experienced without the other. They are both transitory, and this can be discovered through our own experience.

As the knots undo, the energies of our body will flow freely; we are free from having to either ignore or think about them. They are felt directly.

There is then a sense of total relief, of alive calm which can be trusted, as the information received through the senses is less and less distorted. Hence, there is less to fear and to defend our image against. Eventually the need to sustain images disappears, for reality is simply what is, and is lived.

* * *

All our relationships exist only through the body. When our bodies are internally wholly felt in relationship with others, there is no distinction between what is happening face to face and what is happening behind our backs.

If we are on stage in relationships, playing out fixed images and roles, then there must be a backstage, in the dark, and we must suffer the consequence—tremendous conflict. To be fully open in relationship means to be completely free of worry, for there is nothing hidden, nothing to be "found out", nothing to defend.

To give up the superficial and trivial levels of communication—wanting to be loved; wanting to play a role whether good or evil; wanting to be admired; being concerned with what others might think or say, and so on—is to be open to the deeper, living levels of the body. These are what guide in meditation and in life. When our attention is brought to these levels, what is blocking their realisation in life will unfold, untie and unknot.

Interlude 1: The body as a teacher

When our senses are open—from the skin through to the mind—and our perceptions clear, the neurosis of either denying our senses or excessively indulging them disappears. Love and wisdom are then possible.

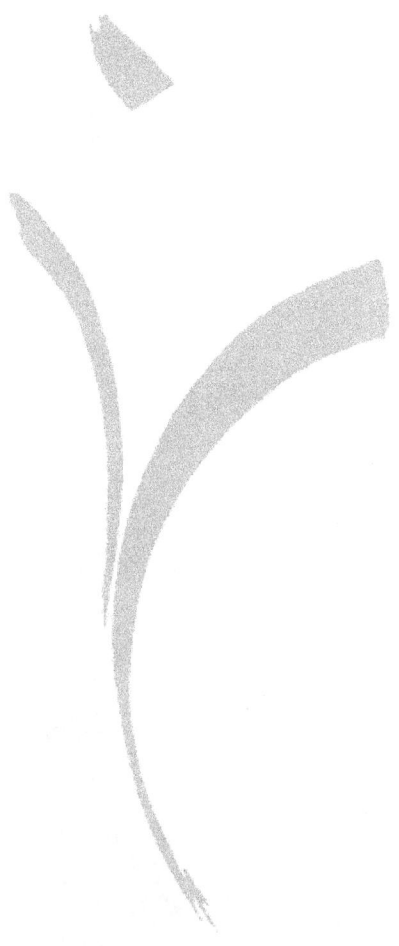

Opening the senses opens the heart.

We all know what we're doing—we just like to pretend we don't.

The path is not the one with big arrows.

CHAPTER 2 | *Why meditation?*

*Becoming aware of and
observing our own minds
leads us to the direct
experience of the ground
of existence: a clear, open,
vibrant, spacious stillness,
beyond separation and
differentiation. From this
experience arise joy,
contentment and well-being.
It is on this basis that we
come to fulfil our lives, to
achieve wisdom and to
know love.*

In observing the way we usually live our lives, it soon becomes evident that conflict is an integral part of nearly every situation we find ourselves in. How do we go beyond this conflict?

Many of us proceed to rearrange the externals of our lives: perhaps changing jobs, looking for different partners in our relationships, seeking new experiences through travel, joining political or idealistic organisations and so on, in the belief that this will remedy the conflict.

We can spend our entire lives doing this and may certainly find short-term benefits, but if we observe others and investigate the history of our civilisation, we find that conflict and frustration are insoluble at this level. We are then left with ourselves, and the question arises as to whether this state of conflict is endemic to human beings.

In the previous chapter the idea was put forward that concepts and ideas about our lives are often at complete variance with what is actually happening, so it is necessary to take this into account when dealing with the question of conflict. What are concepts and ideas? How do they arise? Why do we believe them? Why do we cling to them so tenaciously? What is the alternative?

These are questions which the practice of Insight meditation in particular addresses. Insight meditation is a way of directly experiencing the nature of the mind or consciousness, and its contents. This includes the matrix of all the images, concepts and thoughts that we perceive as our minds, and the images and thoughts themselves. It is then possible to develop clear insight into the way thoughts and images are conditioned, and see beyond them.

This frees us from the confusion generated by what we think we are or should be and enables us, through insight, to integrate all the physical, emotional and mental aspects of our lives. While these aspects are not integrated they are split and so actions, feelings and thoughts may occur without awareness or any unifying intention, thus giving rise to conflict and pain.

The basis of all meditation work is experiential, not conceptual. Identifying ourselves and reality with preconceptions, either inherited or instilled through conviction, creates problems when we attempt to know and to live, because preconceptions are looked upon as a foundation and the acquired knowledge has no basis in experience.

This causes immense confusion because we are not concepts; neither are others, nor is any other form of life. To achieve an understanding of life on this basis is ultimately impossible. We are living, and therefore in a constant state of movement and change.

No phenomenon is stable, independent or permanent. Everything exists interdependently. Therefore a concept, in attempting to name an entity, can only be partially true at best. It cannot be equated with a living, changing organism.

*   *   *

Meditation begins where concepts leave off, not by denying them but by recognising their limitations—their function is to deal with limits, to define. Meditation is a process of perceiving directly, on the understanding that life cannot be known conceptually, but can only be directly experienced. Thus the basis of meditation is direct experience gained through constant observation, unobstructed by preconceptions, thoughts, images and conflicting emotions.

Once this is achieved and recognised, communication becomes effortless, for we are then free to value and use concepts for what they are. We are not driven by our attempts to cling to them nor are we obliged to believe them. To search for concepts divorced from experience is an attempt to fit life into a mould and can only lead to stagnation.

Seeing directly involves not clinging to preconceptions and identities. It is not possible to cease clinging to preconceptions if they are not seen and their limitations are not understood, for until they are seen we will continue to believe them.

Clear thinking is essential for meditation, because the direct experience of meditation needs to be tested through reason in order to be brought to a clearly formulated insight. Direct experience is a creative act, and reason is the faculty which harmonises this with the cultural structures through which we communicate.

The understanding thus derived can be applied to and integrated into our lives. Meditating means balancing: intuition with clear thought, feeling with knowledge, and contemplation with action; conflict cannot be resolved through negations or through one-sidedly affirming one or other of our faculties.

Meditation is a way of going beyond all the forms of perception—sensing, feeling, thinking and intuition—to experience the calm, clear awareness which is the essence of all perception. This awareness or open intelligence is the basis of consciousness. When it is directly experienced, there is no longer any need to identify with or be dependent on a particular form of perception in order to see what is happening.

This means that instead of only one or two forms of perception operating clearly and always being accompanied by the obscuring shadow of the others, all of them will be clear—clear sensing, feeling, thinking and intuition—as the basis from which they derive, clear awareness, is recognised.

* * *

The practice of meditation is the practice of bringing the mind to a state of total absorption in whatever object is chosen. This way of achieving concentration is very different from the usual idea associated with concentration–the act of forcing the mind to come to grips with and tackle a problem. Absorbed concentration is allowing the mind to rest gently on an object in an open, receptive state, just observing or noticing, until there is nothing at all obscuring the object.

In this state there is no separation or differentiation between the mind and its object, and this gives rise to a deep-seated calm. This happens naturally in many situations, for example when reading or at the cinema. However, in meditation practice, the foundation of calm is cultivated and used as a basis for the mind to come effortlessly to one-pointed focus, so that there is a very clear, alert state of awareness.

This state is then developed for the work of insight. It is the general lack of calm in everyday life which prohibits us from developing it. Therefore, the first efforts made in this work are put into bringing the body and emotions to an alive, calm state.

When we are truly absorbed we find that, quite naturally, bliss and joy arise. These are the signs of healing within the body and mind, for they arise when physical and mental knots are released. They are therefore a reference to be used in life because they indicate the basic feeling tone of healthy, clear emotions and states of mind.

Meditation, like all culturally transmitted practices, has its traditions. To try and avoid tradition, or to try to live without it, is foolish, as we are embedded in it. However, we do not need to be its slaves, or simply believe or repeat it. In order to free ourselves from tradition, we need to pick it up, understand it, and be aware of its limitations.

Therefore it is important to understand that rituals, symbols, organisations and so on, are not meditation itself. They are simply images or representations of meditation experiences, or pointers to those experiences. The living, flowing, constant, ancient tradition of meditation is *direct, individual experience*. Everything else is an embellishment of this and can become an encrustation or a hindrance.

For us in the West to take over unquestioningly whole systems of meditation from the East is basically a waste of time. However, there is much that is extremely valuable and which can be adapted to our particular needs.

It is necessary to go directly to and understand the essence of all meditation work. This is the willingness to accept ourselves and to open up and explore inner experience. All methods and practices are designed to assist and sustain this process, for naturally, as with any other work, it is possible to go astray and fool ourselves.

There is nothing intrinsically dangerous in the practice of Insight meditation; however, if we do it with a fixed idea of what should or should not happen, or of what we aim to get out of it, we are obviously headed for trouble, because one of the main functions of meditation is to cut through all preconceptions and fixed ideas. This means seeing ourselves as we actually are, not as we think we ought to be or would like to be.

Working with a guide or teacher and using certain practices enables us to build and understand the foundations upon which all insight is based, and to test the insight when it arises. This entails establishing the calm, healthy state of body, emotions and mind which are essential for any meditation work to come to fruition. And, of course, that takes time.

*   *   *

Meditation is not a rejection of suffering. It is impossible to reject suffering. The price of existence is constant struggle. We might try to blame others for this—parents, politics and so on—or we might try to blame ourselves. We might try and search for the special reasons why it should be us who are suffering. We might try to avoid it and pretend that it is not happening, or we might try to exaggerate and worship it in order to attract a saviour of some kind or another. All of these attempts ultimately achieve only frustration, for they are grounded in wanting and fear.

The only thing which can be done is to face the fact of suffering. Of course this is appalling. No-one is exempt from the pain of both physical and mental disease, senility and death, and the apparent futility of it all.

Meditation is a way of establishing the calm and clarity to face suffering and struggle in order to penetrate right through them. This is what transcendence means: not to float over or avoid something, but to penetrate right through and go beyond it. We can only do this for ourselves, individually, in our own lives here and now.

Through the work of meditation we can penetrate the whole question of suffering and emotional conflict in order to come to the root of the problem and eradicate it. This root is self-will—"my way, my life, my pain, my pleasure, my desire, my fear"—the process of identification. It can only be maintained through a state of confusion and by completely ignoring a great deal of the consequences of our behaviour. This results in a very superficial and partial view of life.

By observing closely what appears simply to happen to us we are able to see, on a much deeper level, a balance operating in our lives between our actions and their consequences. There is no need then for hysteria, depression or boredom, all of which are interdependent and are the products of deliberately or unknowingly ignoring certain aspects of our lives. It becomes possible to see directly that the way we view life shapes what happens to us in our lives.

When the totality of our actions and their consequences is seen, there is no longer any need to pretend to ourselves that we don't know why this or that should happen to us, nor any need to manipulate situations by trying to seduce and control others. There is no need to convince ourselves that our problems are special or different—"my way" is seen for the superficial nonsense that it is. The qualities of our individual lives are then free to become apparent.

*   *   *

To penetrate and transcend superficial and partial views of life brings us to a point of equilibrium and equanimity; a much deeper view and realisation of actuality. At this level it is seen that nothing and nobody exists as a separate phenomenon. Everything is insubstantial and interdependent. There is nothing and no-one separate from our own awareness, nor can we draw lasting happiness or satisfaction from them.

Becoming aware of and observing our own minds lead us to the direct experience of the ground of existence: a clear, open, vibrant, spacious stillness, beyond separation and differentiation. From this experience arise joy, contentment and well-being. It is on this basis that we come to fulfil our lives, to achieve wisdom and to know love.

When we start to crave

we have lost contact with our own heart.

Opening to and accepting inner solitude entail facing the unknown—giving up and letting go of everything we think we know. It leads to the experience of a cool, peaceful, open spaciousness which pervades both the mind and body.

This quality is in total contrast to the cluttered state of endless chatter, usually generating a great deal of heat and conflict, which we invariably associate with our minds. Unwatched and generally unseen, this is the living force behind our lives. It is this which gives us our identity and which then forces us to play the roles and to seek the situations which will confirm and sustain it.

Solitude does not necessarily mean always being alone, for whether we are on our own or in a crowd, the mental conversations continue and can actually generate a feeling of desperate loneliness. This is the antithesis of true solitude.

It is through turning towards and facing our own emotions and minds that solitude and peace develop. For then we start to look behind the scenes, at the ropes and machinery which are propping up our image of ourselves.

The first consequence of this is that while living and relating with others, we do not need to use them to play out and fulfill our inner dialogues. As long as these dialogues are ignored, we are destined to attempt to use others to play them out. But when they are brought to awareness and questioned, the desire to sustain our identity by controlling others dissolves.

*   *   *

Ceasing to ignore emotions and inner conversations is the beginning of letting go of them. This letting go is the essence of inner peace—of freeing ourselves from the cramped, crowded and busy emotional and mental space we live in.

Attempting to come to terms with, to control, to resolve or to deal with what we see as our personal emotional and mental problems, is simply to confirm and sustain the states of mind which are familiar to us. This means that we can continue to ignore the mindstates themselves while busying ourselves with the apparent problems, and thus leave the clutter as it is while making it appear important.

This leaves our identity untouched. The only way to clear these states is to watch them in a calm, receptive way and see what arises. Watching them, bringing them to awareness, will reveal them directly for what they are. There is then no mystery, aura or hidden power around them.

It will be seen that they change and dissolve of their own accord because they cannot do anything else. Then the gaps between them will be revealed, and these gaps are the space of solitude.

If we are prepared to face and watch the conflicts of our own minds instead of being driven by them into some form of distraction, we will always come to this point: to the gaps—the spaces—between the thoughts and images.

It will become evident that no problem is unique or personal, but that what we suffer is simply what every human being suffers. In experiencing the spaces in the mind, conflict will be seen to come from a lack of perspective—from not seeing that thoughts and images can only exist in relation to the space which is their matrix, and that they, too, are ultimately spacious and open.

*   *   *

Becoming aware of this space, feeling and understanding it, is therefore the way out of conflict. Inner space is the same as the space in which clouds and weather patterns come and go. Believing that thoughts and images make up the whole of our minds is the same as believing that there are only clouds and no space surrounding the earth.

This space is the opening to a feeling for others and the whole of life, for it is the matrix of consciousness common to every sentient life-form.

Through turning and facing our own solitude, it is possible to come to a feeling of fulfilment and completion. In experiencing the space of consciousness, we experience our common ground with all life and the clear, open, shimmering silence which balances and permeates our thoughts and emotions.

Only from the depth of our being can we know happiness and contentment.

Inner solitude means letting go of all the attachments we usually sustain in the mind and accepting its lasting openness. Through this arises the realisation that there is no lasting satisfaction or happiness to be found outside ourselves.

Our energies can then be contained, which results in our lives being contented.

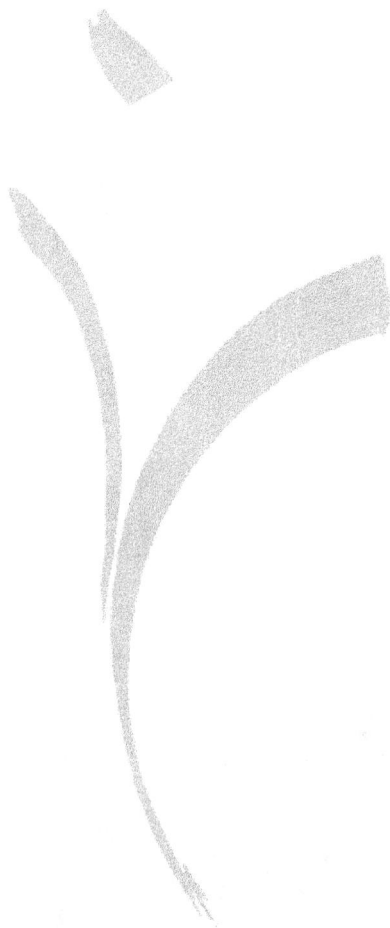

Do not identify with thoughts—they are simply
what they are.
Recognise this and let them come and go.

To cling is to suffer.

To let go and dissolve is to experience bliss.

3 | *Preparation—simplifying the life*

> *Meditating is a touching*
> *of the earth; a touching*
> *of the core of our own being.*
> *It opens us to the experience*
> *of true relaxation: a peaceful,*
> *clear, fulfilling experience*
> *where we learn to nourish*
> *ourselves.*

When beginning meditation, the first prerequisite is space in your life: a time and a place in which it is possible to meditate. This involves simplifying your life, creating space for meditation, and facing one of the fundamental areas of confusion.

A very clear distinction needs to be made between what we actually need and what we think we want—a sorting out of priorities. Our lives are finite. We can either accept this and value our lives, harness our energies in order to penetrate and transcend conflict and come to know happiness, or we can attempt to ignore it.

Needs and wants

Material requirements for maintaining the body are relatively simple: food, clothing, shelter and medicine. All that is necessary is what is adequate for good health and a reasonable level of physical comfort. For these we are interdependent. Even though the idea of physical independence might be pleasant to entertain (the "tropical island" fantasy), the actual reality of the intense labour involved would be daunting, and our total dependence on the earth would need to be acknowledged.

It has been a great achievement of the human race, and particularly of our own culture, to be able to supply the requirements of the body reasonably effortlessly. Organisation and machinery have made physical prosperity possible on a fairly large scale. Problems arise because, having achieved this, nobody seems to know what to do with it, except to go on doing it.

Money then, instead of being viewed simply as a means for supplying our needs, becomes an obsession and there is never enough, even though we might have vast quantities of it. Money, the symbol of wealth, has displaced true wealth, which is material well-being and the freedom to learn. Anticipation has become valued over fulfilment; preoccupation with the security of the future over the actuality of the present; abstraction over reality.

This sort of confusion arises because once physical survival is assured, all kinds of psychological illusions start to be projected onto the physical needs. We often believe that material prosperity is the universal remedy for all problems; however, our culture is finding that this is not so. Once material ease is achieved, psychological disturbances start to manifest, as there is nothing to hinder them or channel them into.

To confuse the physical and the psychological is to create a great deal of conflict and pain. It would be foolish to condemn material achievements; however, it is important to question the insistence on quantity and greed to the exclusion of quality and generosity. Any form of behaviour which is clung to once it has served its purpose becomes destructive, and conspicuous consumption is certainly destructive.

Simplifying the life at the physical level, then, is very important, for until this is achieved it is impossible to see clearly. To deny or starve ourselves is not simplicity and is just as foolish as indulging ourselves. We therefore need a means of livelihood as this is the way our culture operates. For many who have started to consider meditating, this will already have been achieved; however, it is important to note that the whole question of a job or career is completely different when viewed from the perspective of meditation.

When contemplating or entering a career we have many motives, hopes, fears and ambitions, because careers are presented as almost the entire purpose of life. Many people work hard and succeed in fulfilling their ambitions, only to find that it all becomes completely meaningless.

They might then decide to change careers and start again, or drop out and try a new lifestyle. Regardless, they have the opportunity to see that what they have experienced is true: it is meaningless. No matter how hard we work to fulfil desires—and ambition is one of them—they are insatiable.

This is where the problem ceases to become physical and becomes psychological. We need to see that wanting, or craving, is an emotion to which everyone is subject, and that there is no way it can be physically fulfilled. To try and fulfil our cravings is fruitless, for it involves being bound to pleasure and pain; setting up the insatiable, infinite cycle of trying to sustain pleasure and avoid pain.

Pleasure and pain are inseparable; they are interdependent, only having meaning in relation to each other. Pleasure is impermanent, so when it ceases we experience pain. To crave something is painful, to get it is pleasurable, to lose it is painful, and to not get it and be stuck with what we don't want is also painful.

This is why people find it hard to admit they have had enough, for it means facing the question of craving. Choosing pleasure and trying to avoid pain is an impossible situation to maintain simply because they are two sides of the same coin—craving: to want and to not want. This is not to deny pleasure, only to point out that neither is physical pleasure its highest form—the state of meditative absorption is a state of bliss far surpassing physical pleasure—nor is any pleasure permanent or able to give lasting satisfaction.

Going beyond pleasure and pain, which means not attempting to indulge or deny them but accepting them for what they are, is a state of balance and well-being which is lasting and fulfilling. Simplifying the life then, entails being prepared to face desire, and realising that there is no way in which it can be materially fulfilled.

Vocation

When greed is not glorified, it is possible to completely change our attitude to work. Instead of seeing work as either the fulfilment of our life's purpose or the evil necessity which provides for greater and greater pleasures, it can become firstly, the means of providing material necessities, and secondly, a means of communicating with others; of giving to them.

This changes our attitude from one of wanting to one of giving. The way then opens up to doing what interests us, what we love. It requires forgetting fashion, the dictates of parents and peers, and seeing what really does interest us. This is the meaning of vocation.

It is possible this might involve accepting a lower status and salary; however, it will also entail less time having to be spent at work, as it becomes simply one of the facets of our life. Our attitude to work is then considerably simplified as the confusion surrounding its purpose is eliminated.

This establishes a good physical basis in our life. Instead of despising, fearing or being desperately ambitious about work, it can become what all real work is: joyful, interesting and reasonably effortless. As we become honest about this level of our lives and don't look to it for what it can't give, we have the time and energy to balance our lives and to support the practice of meditation in our lives.

Refuge

Meditation work begins by re-orienting the mind: moving the focus from outer distractions and preoccupations towards observing our own lives. This is done in two ways: by developing a feeling for inner space or for the depth of our own being, and by establishing a dialogue with a guide or teacher.

It is not often that we are truly calm and confident within ourselves, having a feeling of self worth and a real respect for our own lives. This is because we perceive our individuality on a very superficial level, and are used to relating to others at that level. In fact, we are encouraged to do so.

Building a dialogue with a meditation teacher or guide means relating with someone else beyond the casual, superficial levels with which we are familiar, for it engages every level of our being. It is a dialogue in which every habit, preconceived idea and image of ourselves is questioned.

The dialogue is pointing constantly to the depth of our being;

the potential for clear, all-embracing awareness which opens up an understanding of and feeling for the totality of our being. It is this inner silence which can be trusted and in which we can take refuge; this is the source of happiness and fulfilment.

Naturally, this exposes all the fears involved with giving up what we think we are, and the function of a dialogue with a teacher is for these fears to transmute to respect. Respect for other living beings, respect for the work being done, and respect for our own lives. This in turn will gradually transmute to awe or wonder as we begin to view life from this perspective, and will eventually turn into a state of complete openness and clarity.

The practice of meditation is not for solving what are perceived as personal emotional or mental problems. If we still view ourselves in this way, it means that we are not yet ready to face the totality of the question of emotional conflict.

Psychological problems are conceived personally and are therefore still in the realm of dialoguing with the image we have of ourselves. It is only when we are prepared to let go of these levels of dialogue that the practice of Insight meditation can be fruitful. If there is a need for psychotherapy, it is therefore much healthier and more honest to visit a psychotherapist.

Any dialogue with a teacher can only be sustained on a basis of trust—of knowing we have chosen this dialogue. As we test our work with the teacher through our reason, intuition, senses and feelings, it leads us to realise our inner confidence and to bring this into all aspects of our lives, so that we are able to relate with life at all levels. The totality of our being can then be brought to realisation in our lives.

Everyone, often without realising it, seeks safety in their family, or in power, their job, their possessions, money, or fame for example. However, no meaningful refuge can ultimately be taken in parents, relatives, dependents, institutions, wealth, career and so on, for all of these depend on conditioned, conventional relationships and defined roles, and so lead us away from experiencing our innate wholeness. It is only through coming to understand and through developing a feeling for the depth of our own being, that a deep-seated trust and confidence in our lives is possible.

Ethics

In observing our lives, we will come to notice the relationship which exists between our actions and their consequences. The awareness of this relationship forms the basis of ethical behaviour; ethical actions are those which are skilful and have fruitful consequences; neither wasteful nor destructive.

To imagine that what happens to us in life is either a reward or a punishment for good or bad behaviour, or is the fault of somebody or something else, is to obscure our states of mind, rendering it impossible to see them. The question of action, of what we do and how it is motivated, is fundamental to the practice of meditation, and so it is essential to observe carefully which of our actions are effective and which are not.

We will then be able to see that what happens to us is the direct result of what we do and of how we view life. If we see others as threatening to our existence and way of life, eventually this is exactly how they will appear to behave. If we are prepared to listen to others and to treat them as human beings rather than objects requiring manipulation, we will find that life becomes more open for us—freer and more effortless.

If we attempt to walk through a city with our eyes closed and our ears blocked, it is fairly probable that we will sustain a certain amount of physical damage. Therefore, it is wise to keep our senses alert and open, and not be surprised when dull, deadened, drugged, overloaded or overindulged senses, and the consequent state of unawareness, lead to unfortunate situations. These are not a punishment for sinful behaviour, but simply the result of a confused, unaware state of mind.

One of the factors which can hinder seeing this process clearly is that occasionally there can be a considerable time delay between an action and its consequence. This occurs mainly because we are in some ways cushioned from the direct results of our actions by relationships and social institutions.

For example, someone who is accident prone might not realise that, if left alone, their state of unawareness would lead to death, as they are often saved by friends and emergency services. It is, however, ultimately impossible to save anyone from the consequences of their actions, and unless the warnings of accidents are heeded and watchfulness cultivated, the inevitable distressing results will occur.

It is an overriding state of confusion which hinders the clear seeing of this process. This confusion is often deliberately cultivated for the purpose of not seeing what is being done in order to be able to deny responsibility for it. The hope is that the consequences of actions will either be blamed on others, or that others will take pity on us and look after us.

Relationships with others form an important part of our lives, and here too, it is necessary to become aware of and watch habitual patterns which can be unskilful and unhealthy, leading to painful situations. Perhaps the simplest way of coming to see them and let go of them is to take to heart the old Zen saying—*After eating, wash your own bowl.*

More often than not, taking refuge in others means wanting them to look after us, which is ultimately an impossible situation to fulfil. In order, therefore, to clear a lot of confusion out of our lives it is necessary to take on the training of cleaning up after ourselves, until this becomes effortless.

One common habitual pattern is leaving messages for others to find—what could be called the "throw-away" mentality. Our disposable, consumer culture encourages this so that someone else is required to clean up or dispose of what we throw away. It's a way of being noticed and of expressing a sense of power.

Many relationships are built on this principle. Unfortunately, it is not realised that if we leave things for others to find and clean up or return, we either become dependent on them or we force them into being dependent on us. Thus there is a great deal which must remain unspoken, hidden with confusion and repressed—all of which will emerge painfully later on.

Using others for our pleasure is a way of trying to avoid our own emotions, and is also an attempt to get others to clean up after us. This is using others as an emotional handkerchief. The result of this is an eventual alienation from others, leading to self-pity and depression.

In relationships, it is far wiser to ground dialogue in mutual respect, where it is understood that it is impossible to take on responsibility for another's life, and where each is responsible for his or her own life. Relationships can then be free from fantasy and based on mutual interest, and on this basis it is possible to develop a sense of real worth in, and a caring for our own life and the lives of others. The basis of all ethics then, is wise action: being mindful and honest in what we do and say, and accepting the consequences.

Clearing a space

In coming to the actual practice of meditation there needs to be a space in which to work: a room where we can be alone, which is as clean and tidy as possible, and in which the air is fresh. It is also necessary to make sure that our body and clothes are clean.

These are very simple things; however, the immediate environment feeds information to the mind, and it will all be read out in meditation. If the environment is cluttered and chaotic, this will directly affect the meditation practice, and will lead to confused, painful states of mind, and a waste of time and effort.

Clearing a space also involves ensuring that there is time in which to meditate. This entails gently letting go of the ways for simply passing time which have been built up in our lives, such as habitual socialising.

The bodily posture is also important, for states of mind and postures are interdependent. The state of mind generated in meditation can be determined and fed by a particular or habitual posture. Therefore the posture needs to be stable, comfortable, calm and alert.

All meditation practice rests on a state of balanced calm. This is attained through establishing a relaxed, observant and healthy life.

Beginning meditating

Initially, ten minutes per day is sufficient to establish the practice of meditation. This can gradually be increased to half an hour per session and eventually to one hour, which is the maximum time given to any session of meditation as our natural concentration span is about fifty minutes or so.

It is very important that there is no attempt to force meditating, or to push the time of the session beyond where it is comfortable. Therefore, short frequent sessions are much better and ultimately more productive than longer ones—tired and dull states of mind are not conducive to meditation.

When meditating is consistently effortless and agreeable, it is possible to increase the time span comfortably: from ten to twenty minutes, then to half an hour, to forty minutes, to one hour. However, it is important to gauge ourselves and to stop while still fresh; then it will always be pleasant to return to the practice, and interest will be maintained.

The best times for meditating are first thing in the morning and around sunset. However, if this is not possible, it is simply a matter of arranging ten minutes somewhere in the daily schedule. Allowing one day per week without formal meditation allows room for informal meditation practices, for integrating what has been experienced, for results to arise spontaneously, for keeping the practice fresh, and for incorporating any rebellious tendencies.

There are two sitting postures for formal practice: one in a chair, the other on the floor. It is essential to feel comfortable while meditating, so there is no need to force the body into postures which are painful. This becomes self-defeating.

As most of us are used to sitting in chairs, this is the posture most people find comfortable. For sitting in a chair, a straight-backed, padded chair (or armchair) is best, so that it will support the spine in a straight position. The knees are held at right angles and well apart so that the stomach can relax, and the feet are flat on the floor.

For sitting on the floor it is best to sit on a fairly high cushion with the legs crossed, so that the knees are on the floor. This means the buttocks are higher than the knees. Any way of crossing the legs is fine, as long as it is comfortable—either full or half lotus (both feet on the thighs, or one foot only), or with one foot in front of the other, or with the feet loosely crossed. Stability is achieved by resting on the buttocks and both knees. If it is physically impossible to place both knees on the floor, stability and a straight spine can be achieved by resting the back against a wall. Or you might prefer to use a meditation stool which enables you to sit comfortably on the floor.

Whether you are sitting in a chair or on the floor, the spine needs to be held comfortably erect, neither slumped nor rigid. The hands are rested on the thighs, or together in the lap just below the navel, with the right on top of the left, the palms facing upwards, and the thumbs gently touching. The belly is relaxed, and the chin pulled in slightly to open the back of the neck. The eyes are held half-open and focussed gently in front while looking slightly down, or if it is more comfortable in the beginning, closed. The mouth is closed with the jaw relaxed. For developing calm the tongue can be relaxed with the tip resting below the bottom teeth.

Four ideas for contemplation

There are four themes for reflection which are traditionally given at the beginning of the practice of meditation. These are preparatory reflections to set the motivation for the work and help re-orient the mind.

Valuing our life

The first is to reflect on the value of human life and on the value of our own lives in particular. Compared with other forms of life, human beings are in a minority on this planet, and to have a life where material needs are fulfilled, where there is political freedom, where the body and mind are whole and healthy, where you have the opportunity for education, and the inclination, opportunity and time to practise meditation, is comparatively very rare. Therefore, it is important to value this life and not waste it.

Accepting the reality of death

The second is to reflect on death. Everything is impermanent. Nobody is exempt from death; it can come at any time and at the time of death, nobody can help or save us. We are then subject to our own minds and the habits which have been established in them during our lives.

The consequences of actions

The third is the reflection on action and the law of cause and effect. Whatever actions we take in this life, we will eventually reap their consequences. It is important, therefore, to recognise and cultivate healthy actions and to recognise and relinquish unhealthy ones.

Living with mindfulness

The fourth reflection is to contemplate the disadvantages of wandering blindly through life, attempting to grasp at pleasure and avoid pain. Its purpose is to constantly remind ourselves to not fall into a semi-hypnotic state whenever we are relaxed and comfortable.

It's useful to keep in mind that none of us is exempt from the experience of pain in our lives. It can come through sickness and old age, through the fact that everything changes and that all pleasant experiences eventually come to an end, and that no matter how good it gets, we all experience an underlying frustration and dissatisfaction which keep goading us to want more and more.

Continually bringing these ideas to mind helps prepare the way for simplifying the life, and establishing and sustaining the practice of meditation in our lives.

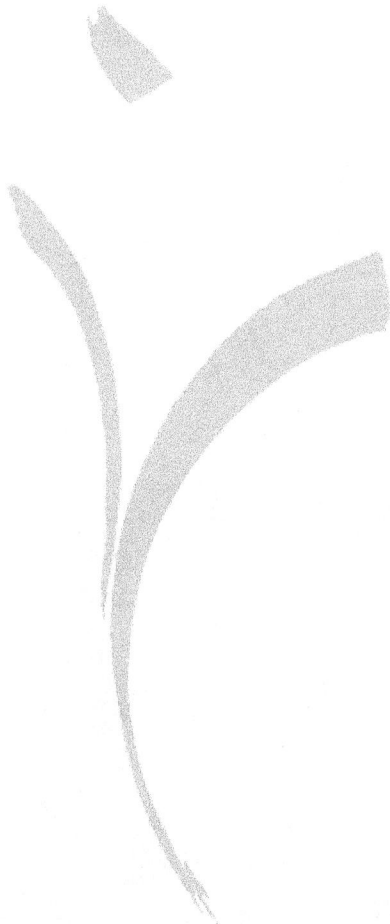

When we make the cosmos cosmetic,

we become comatose.

Work is the sign of friendship

To work is to find and fulfill our vocation—and ultimately to come to work on ourselves; to know ourselves totally. This means facing in ourselves all the hopes and fears to which everyone is subject, and to free ourselves from all fixed concepts and preconceived ideas. This is the work of meditation.

Work is a constant question.

To love is to open to the deepest and widest form of desire, for love is infinite and ultimately without an object. It is love which draws us to find our true vocation.

True kindness is to work because it is the fruit of this work which will feed ourselves and others—it is sharing.

All religions have sold the lie of liberation without work: the lie that either someone has done the work for all, or that someone else is doing it, and all we need to do is to believe, to have faith. This is most destructive, for it distracts us from facing the conflict that exists in ourselves and renders us impotent to do anything about it.

The basis of all existence is conflict—the constant dialogue between hope and fear. Each of us must face this dialogue within ourselves, and go beyond its projections. The only foundation on which this can be done is work—the work of taking on that struggle totally, and seeing it. This means being prepared to face it and not expecting or hoping that someone else will save us from it, which is an impossible thing to do.

*   *   *

It is through taking on our own work and living our own conflict totally that we will come to experience love, and open ourselves to total desire without projection. When we experience this we understand the difference between desire which is based on trying to repeat something that happened before or on fulfilling an idea we have in our head, and desire which is related to the reality of our bodies, our lives and what is happening around us.

In the first instance the desire is so focused on the idea of what we want that it completely disconnects us from reality. It is based on a thought about something, and is not based on what is actually happening or the people with whom we are communicating. When our desire is based on real needs and is connected to the reality of our bodies, it is related to the people and situations we are actually living with.

Opening ourselves to the totality of desire will bring us to see that unhealthy desire, or craving, is at the root of all conflict—and it is through seeing this directly that there is liberation from craving, fear and frustration.

When craving—that insatiable yearning which comes from desiring the idea of something rather than relating to something real—is seen directly, without distraction, there is nothing more to want. The mind has faced totally the source of all its searching and seeking, and in doing that, there cannot be any differentiation between what is searching and the object it is seeking.

Craving can only exist when the whole mind is not seen. When it is seen totally, the chain of craving is broken because there is no secret; nothing hidden; nothing to look for and therefore nothing to fear.

In fulfilling our vocation, we are living the way to liberation. This example is what will feed others, for it is a living, testable, provable action: a statement that the conflict inherent in life *can* be faced. It is a statement that everybody can see for themselves, and it frees the way for true dialogue—dialogue based on action. When people meet and are prepared to dialogue on this basis, then there is friendship.

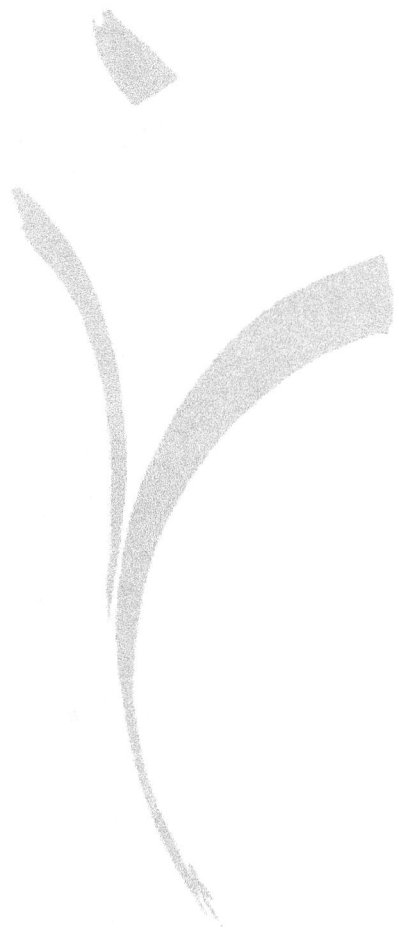

Wanting + Fear = Frustration.

There is no competition—everyone dies.

It is impossible to live without commitment—

we are committed to breathing.

4 | *Foundation—sustaining the question*

This is the only way to see clearly—to cultivate a calm, receptive patience and allow things to come to us of their own accord, for as soon as we grasp at something we miss it.

Because we succumb all too easily to an immediate answer; because we invariably set goals—either of success or failure—and try to attain them as quickly as possible; because we strive; there is a need for a body of practices which will carry us through and beyond goals, answers and aims, until we are able, in fact are quite content, to simply remain with the question.

Grasping at judgements and answers is the greatest hindrance to seeing clearly, and learning to give this up brings us face to face with our basic insecurity and anxiety; for we do not like to admit that we do not know.

However, the only security there is, is letting go of all our preconceptions, and learning to see and experience directly and clearly. Therefore the foundation of Insight meditation is the practice of unknowing: of giving up all that we think we know; of not grabbing or grasping at new and recognisable answers; of learning to sustain the state of question.

This is the only way to see clearly—to cultivate a calm, receptive patience and allow things to come to us of their own accord, for as soon as we grasp at something we miss it. We need to learn to defer judgement and to observe and investigate what is right in front of us and what we are involved in, until we have a feeling for all its aspects; until our view is complete and not partial.

Because of fixed ideas and set habit patterns, very rarely does anyone see all the options available in any particular situation. Life then feels as though it is inevitably being driven in a given direction. But this need not be so: it only happens because of an inability to defer judgement and allow the options to become apparent. This stems from habitually grasping at what is immediately recognisable. The response then, is not to what actually is but to a remembered image of past experience.

Insight cannot be grasped, pushed or forced into happening. It arises naturally when the circumstances are conducive. The work is in creating these circumstances, in letting go of all that we think we are, should be, might become, or plan to do, and allowing the mind to rest and settle, freeing it from all the grasping and goal orientation with which it is usually occupied. We are then prepared, and so are able to recognise insight when it arises.

The most difficult thing to do is to be alone and to sit still, not attempting to do anything. This is where meditation practices from the East are invaluable, for they give us something to do while we are learning to be still. At the same time they are continually directing the mind to the pertinent questions, so that we learn to recognise and sustain these questions.

The practices outlined here are adapted from the Mahamudra meditation tradition of the Tibetan Karma Kargyu lineage in such a way that their essence and the principles they embody can be used effectively in Western life. Although they are not essential to the development of calm and concentration and insight, and are part of the body of practices known as Tantra, they are included because they have always been an integral part of Mahamudra. Their purpose is to provide the foundation for integrating the realisations of insight into our lives.

Each practice is designed to bring the mind to a completely open state while focusing on a particular area of our lives, until a "sign" as it is traditionally termed, or an insight, arises, leading to a depth understanding in that area. This involves dialogue with a guide or teacher—someone who has gone before—in order to confirm the validity of these insights, thereby sorting out at the basic preliminary level what is complete and what is only partial. Developing a feeling for and an understanding of insight at this level means that the more subtle levels of the practice will be able to flow with confidence and relative ease.

As has been pointed out, the work of foundation is in sustaining and focussing question; in creating the circumstances in our lives which are conducive to the arising of insight and which prepare us for recognising insight when it arises; in allowing the insight to deepen and in trusting it.

The work is also an act of compassion, both toward ourselves and others. For through it we have the opportunity to understand our lives and conditioning completely—our own bodies. Then the clarity of insight can be fully integrated into our lives on all levels: physically, emotionally and mentally.

It can then be communicated, not just through speaking but through living, and our life can be an example of true freedom. Not licence to do what we want, but complete freedom from wanting itself. Until there is total freedom from our cravings there is always an element of confusion no matter how subtle, for our viewing is still selective and consequently not total. It is to this level of clarity and clear seeing that Insight meditation is addressed.

Nobody really comes to understand through what is said, but

through communicating with someone who has directly experienced: who is the experience. They can then feel it. This is what compassion means—communication which can be felt, which derives from a feeling with and for others.

It is at the fundamental level of foundation work that this understanding is developed. This work is to come to understand our own conflict and thereby the conflict of others. It is facile to consider that there is no need to work: life is work, we are working anyway. Whether we like it or not the body keeps eating, defecating, breathing and so on.

The practice of meditation is the union of insight and compassion. The function of a guide is not to say what the realisation is, but to point the way so that each individual might come to experience truth and love directly in his or her own life. Because realisation is direct experience it is beyond concepts, and is therefore ultimately impossible to communicate through concepts. The only way to free ourselves from conflict and confusion is to do it for ourselves, in our own lives.

*   *   *

The foundation practices involve repetition on a large scale: repetition of practices involving the body, the emotions, the mind and the integration of all three. Each practice is repeated 100,000 times, or until the sign arises. The original text actually says just to do a large number until the sign arises, so there is no need to be too fussy about the number itself. It is necessary to understand that there is no such thing as direct repetition, but constant variation.

This work then, is a letting go, a cleaning out of all fixations so that our focus moves away from goals, both inner and outer, to just seeing what we are actually doing at the moment we are doing it, clearly and simply, and understanding it.

The scale of the work is large, for a common attitude to work is to get rid of it as quickly as possible in order to get onto something "real", which usually means a habitual fantasy we wish to indulge. There is a vast difference between doing something and trying to get rid of it: just doing what is there to be done patiently, realising that there is no competition, no prizes, no applause, no rush, and nothing better to do. Each activity and each action has its own quality.

This work is learning about ourselves and is done in a relaxed fashion, with interest, so that it becomes a continuum in our life. It is learning to be patient and friendly with ourselves and coming to know all the different aspects of our lives. It involves watching our reactions to the work and learning to feel it internally at a fine and subtle level. *The work itself is the question that we are constantly posing—we simply watch what we do with it.*

The work of foundation is the creation of emotional and mental space in the life. It is the vehicle for disengaging from the compulsive controls in our lives, from all the things we feel compelled to do because we think they are essential for our survival. This entails letting go of them, and allowing them to look after themselves, so that we do not keep maintaining the illusion that we are indispensable in any situation.

From this arises a complete re-orientation, for it becomes evident to us that we are not needed for life to keep going. Then it is possible to learn to sustain inner solitude and so not be emotionally dependent on others or on social situations. We will then be in a position to relate to others enjoyably and in a relaxed way.

There is not an absolutely right way to do these practices. All that needs to be done is to keep them going, allow them to unfold, and observe what we do with them. The observation encompasses every level of our being: our bodies and postures, the attitudes we take to the practices and to the blocks and knots they reveal; to the feelings and sensations involved; to the states of mind which arise; and to the objects we habitually choose to think about; that is, the habitual thoughts, images and inner dialogues which go on in the mind.

There are four foundation practices: prostrations, clearing of emotional and mental states, mandala offering, and integration.

Prostrations

This practice is physical, and although it has an enormous effect on the body, straightening the spine and bringing the body to a fluid and supple state, it is not designed primarily as a physical exercise. It is pointing to a direct understanding of our physical existence. The practice involves prostrating ourselves, full length on the floor, while reciting a mantra. Mantra is a Sanskrit word which derives from *mano* meaning "mind" and *tra* meaning "tool". So it literally means "mind tool" and is a word-symbol used to generate particular feelings and images.

The first thing this practice brings into question is our habitual physical and mental orientation. It is very difficult for someone conditioned in a Western culture to deliberately put his or her head on the ground, except at the beach. The common attitude is to have the head in the future or in books and abstract concepts, and the feet in pollution.

This practice brings us to feel the ground, literally, with the whole body, head included, so that we are putting our heads where our feet are: a complete re-orientation of perspective. By placing our whole body on the floor we can feel and understand how its ground, or foundation, is the earth. Our bodies come from the earth, are nourished by it and eventually return to the earth.

It is essential for understanding ourselves, and developing a feeling for the depth of our being, to learn to listen to the body—allowing it to teach us. Our bodies are the crystallisation of all our past experience; they are our contact with the earth, the vehicle for our lives, and the means for all relationships and communication.

To punish, coddle or try to perfect the body are all attempts at avoiding it. The practice of prostrations is an acceptance of the body; a surrendering of our views of the body and of life, and an opening of ourselves to coming down to earth. This acceptance frees us from creating pollution in our lives, for there is the understanding that what we no longer need, when let go of and given freely, becomes manure for new growth.

Begin a prostration by standing with the hands held in front of the chest, palms touching. Then raise them to the forehead and touch it with the knuckles of the thumbs. At the forehead visualise a white light while reciting the syllable OM. Then place the hands at the throat, where a red light is visualised, while reciting the syllable AH. Finally touch the hands to the heart, where a deep blue light is visualised, while reciting the syllable HUM (pronounced HOONG).

Then prostrate the body, full-length on the floor, with the arms outstretched. One prostration is completed when the body is brought back to the upright position. A folded blanket on the floor for the knees and the upper body, and socks on the hands, can help.

Washing the mind and body—emotional and mental clarity

The second practice uses visualisation and mantra to become aware of the very fine, subtle feelings of our bodies and minds. These are usually perceived as emotions; however, what we normally register as an emotion is very crude in comparison, and it arises when there is a block at this level of perception.

In other words, what we usually call emotions are reactions which occur well after the event when we begin thinking about it. They are therefore inappropriate, and distort our perceptions. In not seeing clearly what actually is, we attempt to approximate our responses to what we think was, or ought to be. Habitual emotions are the registering of the conflict which subsequently arises.

The level of very fine sensing is subtle and intelligent, and enables us to feel immediately what is, both around and within us. It is at this level of awareness that we realise how completely we are embedded in life, for every event around us resonates within us. When we learn to become aware of this, our feelings are undistorted and clear, like a stream flowing freely through us, and a state of well-being and joy arises.

What we experience as desire, fear, anger and frustration are extremely crude distortions of what is occurring at this level, simply because we have no awareness or training in how to register feelings, that is, in how to understand the resonances within our own bodies. Therefore this practice is a washing; a cleansing of the habitual emotions and states of mind which obscure these feelings so that the full range and depth of resonance and feeling can come to awareness—clearly, openly and immediately.

When this happens we discover the foundation of our feelings, the clear, open state of awareness which vibrates through all our senses and our entire body, giving it a sense of luminosity.

A good form of this meditation is to visualise a large sphere of white light above the head. From it flows a stream of clear, milky-white liquid. This enters the body through the top of the head and gradually fills the body, while expelling all accumulated debris and tired, dead, knotted feelings as a dark liquid through the fingers and toes, and as smoke through the pores of the skin. The white liquid overflows the top of the head and washes over the outside of the body, so that the body is completely immersed in and filled with a flowing stream of milky-white liquid. The visualisation is dissolved by bringing the light, and all the liquid, which turns to light, to the heart. The light reduces to a pinpoint of light and disappears.

The mantra is OM VAJRA SATTVA HUM

It is pronounced OM VAHJRAH SUTVAH HOONG

Vajra Sattva means "Diamond Being", and represents the diamond state of consciousness in which the mind is totally open, clear, radiant and fully aware.

Mandala offering

The word *mandala* literally means "mind expansion" (*mano* meaning "mind"). This is exactly what this practice is designed for: to open the mind fully, so that instead of the usual cramped, closed, heavy and busy space in which we habitually conduct our lives, we come to know the open, light, clear and spacious state of mind in which it is possible to live. Therefore, this practice is a way of opening and expanding the mind, focussing on the objects—the thoughts and images—which are usually held within the mind.

The practice is done both physically and mentally, by building up and dissolving a small mandala. Using rice and a clear, shiny metal plate, a mandala is constructed of small symmetrically placed heaps of rice, representing everything we are thinking at that moment. It is then dissolved quickly, and the process immediately repeated. Everything we think and that we think we are, is offered, let go of and given up to the space from which it originally came.

Mandala offering points the way to understanding the nature of the mind, by watching the construction of thoughts and their dissolution. Understanding this enables us to be freed from habitual and obsessive thought patterns, for they are simply the scars of past experience.

It is a physical practice which provides a way of literally playing out how thoughts come and go in the clear, open space of the mind. It's a way of letting go of thoughts so as to see and focus on the spaces between them, and then open up to the foundation of the mind. The two sides of the mind are then able to be seen and known: the moving thoughts, coming and going and the still foundation—clear, open, spacious and, like a mirror, simply reflecting everything.

For this practice, a bag of rice and a small, shiny metal plate are needed. The mandala consists of seven small heaps of rice representing the centre and four quarters of the universe, the sun and the moon.

The heaps of rice are placed in order: firstly at the centre of the plate, then at the four cardinal points, and then on either side of the central heap. The following can be recited once each time you start the practice:

"The ground is purified with scented water and strewn with flowers. On it is placed the centre and four quarters of the universe, the sun and the moon. I offer this for the sake of all."

The plate is then held up, and the mandala dissolved quickly by wiping off all the rice.

The mantra which accompanies this practice is OM VAJRA AH HUM.

This is pronounced OM VAHJRAH AH HOONG.

Once the rhythm is established, each heap of rice can represent whatever thought comes into the mind at the moment. The thought is stated as each heap is placed on the plate.

Integration

The conflict that exists between what we do, say, feel and think is dissolved through recognising the clear, open intelligence common to our senses, feelings, intellect and intuition. In this way, our minds, emotions and bodies can be completely integrated.

Each of the previous practices develops an understanding and feeling for this quality of intelligence at each of these three different levels, moving from the relatively slow level of the physical body through to the extremely quick level of the mind. The mind is so subtle, evanescent and in such a constant state of change, that it is only by starting with the body in this way that we gain insight into the mind. It is then possible to see clearly the relationship between our states of mind, our emotions and our bodies.

The final foundation practice, using visualisation and mantra, points to the state of their integration, where the body and the emotions are calm and alive, and the mind clear, through the understanding of the open nature of mind and its vivid, unobstructed awareness. It points to the realisation of going beyond conflict and confusion in this life in our own bodies, and of the state of warm, calm balance: the realisation of truth and love.

An important aspect of this practice is to create the feeling of re-integrating into our lives what we knew and experienced as children. While maintaining the thinking skills of an adult, meditation provides the tools for re-discovering and integrating the open, absorbed, concentrated wonder of a child. The visualisation represents this integrated state.

Traditionally, this practice is referred to as Guru Yoga; *guru* meaning "one who has heard" and *yoga* meaning "to join". Therefore, this practice is a joining with the guru, with the core of our being, the essence of wisdom. The visualisation is adapted from the Nyingma lineage of the Tibetan tradition.

On a large open flower, on which is a cushion of light, is seated a youthful figure, richly robed and completely at ease in a state of joyful, open, clear awareness, totally free from distraction and conflicting emotions. The quality of this figure is that of childlike, peaceful openness which is totally watchful. The visualisation can either be in front, so that the figure is facing you, or on top of your head.

The mantra is:

OM AH HUM VAJRA GURU PADMA SIDDHI HUM

This is pronounced:

OM AH HOONG VAHJRAH GURU PAYMAY SIDDEE HOONG.

Its meaning is as follows:

Vajra	Knowledge and Skill
Guru	Wisdom
Padma	Compassion
Siddhi	Accomplishment and power
Hum	Integration in the body

Each of these practices lays the foundation for continuous observation: observation of the body, feelings, states of mind and objects of mind. They can be done concurrently and are adapted, through dialogue with a guide or teacher, to suit the requirements of each individual. As mentioned previously, they are not necessary for developing calm and concentration or insight, but are included here because they are an integral part of the Mahamudra tradition. As part of the stream of Tantra they are given before developing calm and insight to help integrate the realisations of meditation into the body. This is why they are so repetitive.

We ignore the gift of love with
our demand for perfection.

One of the most unfortunate misconceptions we hold is that love is something we get from someone else. We are led to believe that it is there for the taking, that it is something we have a right to, and that once we have it, all that is required is to "fall in" or swoon. It is not supposed to take any real effort or understanding on our part and, once obtained, should look after itself.

Assumptions like these are commonly held, and are considered to be obvious truths which do not need to be questioned. Somehow, we do not make the connection that a great deal of personal suffering is due to such assumptions.

The basic feeling behind all the assumptions is that love is something outside ourselves which we need to ingest and is therefore dependent on someone else. It needs to be asked whether this is actually so.

It would be useful to see if this feeling has any basis in actual experience. The one area where it would appear to have some validity is in infancy, for it is certainly true that an infant's overall relationship with her mother is one of ingestion. She is totally dependent on her mother for survival, and the first dialogue with her mother is sucking milk from the breast. At this time she is being held and would experience feelings of warmth, support and a comfortable full stomach.

At first glance, this would appear to be a rather idyllic situation; however, there is a price to be paid. Firstly, the infant is totally dependent on her mother for support and nourishment. Secondly, she has very little mobility and absolutely no control over her environment at all, except possibly through expressing discomfort through noise. Thirdly, there is no choice over who the mother is, and so at the time of feeding, all the odours and emotions of the mother, pleasant and unpleasant, are also ingested.

As the list grows, it is seen that what might appear as a blissful time of life and an effortless way of being fed has its problems, and is far more risky than we are usually prepared to recognise. There seems to be a pull, a yearning in the emotions, to return to this state where everything appears to be given effortlessly. However, when viewed clearly, it must be asked whether the price is worth paying. The main price is that of total dependency and an extremely restricted world, which is true also from the mother's point of view, as her energies are almost totally absorbed by the infant.

*   *   *

So the first dialogue all of us have experienced is one of total dependency on another human being. This involved being fed and perhaps this explains why it seems to be an obvious truth that love is a situation where we are helpless and in which something comes from someone else.

It appears therefore that the basic assumptions about love—something which we have to get and once having obtained "fall into", whereby it will all look after itself—do seem to apply in the situation of being fed in infancy. Does this mean that what we experience as love is synonymous with being fed?

Certainly it has something to do with the feelings associated with being fed, namely fulfilment, contentment, and so on, but as has been stated, in infancy this also necessitates total dependency.

As the child grows and gains a certain amount of independence of movement, her mother does not want to give her breast any more, and although food is still given, it requires much more effort to eat it. Eventually it has to be eaten independently of her mother; a hard lesson for the child. It would seem then, that the price of freedom is loss of love.

*   *   *

If we watch relationships, our own and others, we find that dependency appears to be one of the operating assumptions. Most relationships have a not-so-subtle undercurrent whereby one partner is totally dependent on the other in one area, and the dependency is reciprocated in some other area. For example, one might be dependent financially and the other emotionally, and the reward for dependency in one area is total control in the other.

If one partner, once the relationship has been established, wishes to alter the balance of power in the interests of a little more freedom, there is often an emotional eruption and the relationship breaks down. The price of freedom, under these circumstances, certainly does appear to be the loss of love. That is, if being fed either financially or emotionally is love. The problem is that most of us seem to think so.

If we look a little closer at the situation it starts to resemble more a state of war, or at best an armed truce, rather than love. The well known saying, "All's fair in love and war", bears witness to this. Why is this so?

At her mother's breast the infant is truly dependent, both physically and emotionally. Without this support she would die.

Her mother's feelings of nurture and care are essential for her survival. However, as adults, this is not so. We are quite capable of obtaining our own food, and we have a range of choices when it comes to relating emotionally.

Therefore, the way we relate in the name of love is, more often than not, a complete falsification of the facts. We are playing out with others infantile dialogues which have no ground in reality at all. And we are quite prepared to lie to each other in these dialogues—"Without you, I would die"—in order to sustain the illusion of infant dependency. Perhaps this explains why many people expect that anything which is called love will eventually reveal itself to be a lie or at best a confidence trick.

*   *   *

How is it that these infantile dialogues perpetuate themselves into adulthood? Perhaps it is a matter of education? If so, we need to look at what we are taught about love.

The major doctrine on this subject in Western culture is that God is love; God is the Father and we are His children. If this is so, where does ordinary Dad stand? After trying to be God for a number of centuries, he now seems to be conspicuous by his absence.

The Church has taught that the full experience of love (union with God) can only be revealed after we die. Therefore it is not possible to know love fully in this life, only after death. Traditionally, the Church itself has been presented as the Mother, and has encouraged dependency and belief without question. This confirms the assumption that to move towards freedom or knowledge means loss of mother and love.

In school, the work in class tends to treat love only as a joke, if at all. Outside the classroom, particularly among boys, it is experienced as having a lot to do with sex, and a lot of extremely uncomfortable emotions which no-one else seems to be interested in or even aware of.

The only question left seems to be: Why isn't any of this questioned? Even though love is presented such that we'll lose it as soon as we question it, the case for love as viewed so far seems to be completely lost, so there is nothing more to lose by questioning it. For if we were to return to our mother and demand the breast, there is no certainty that it would be given—more likely than not she would be horrified. And even if it were, there would probably be nothing to drink out of it anyway.

For mothers, the situation would hold none of its former charm or interest. We'd all be too big to hold, we wouldn't smell as nicely as we used to, and we certainly couldn't be controlled or dominated physically.

There doesn't seem to be any sense in not questioning the situation, so perhaps the only reason it is not generally questioned is because everyone is convinced that they know what love is. Certainly many institutions—religious, political and so on, as well as many food manufacturers, fast food outlets, advertising companies and the entertainment industry—benefit considerably from the fact that love is viewed in this way.

*   *   *

The greatest hindrance to knowledge is to think that we know, so it would be an interesting exercise to question each of the assumptions about love and see what fruit this bears. These are firstly: that love is something external that we have to get from someone else. Secondly: that having got it we only have to "fall in" or swoon. And thirdly: that it takes no effort or understanding on our part.

Let us take the last assumption first. One of the fundamental observations we can make about life is that it requires effort. The first breath we draw requires effort. For an infant to assimilate sensory input, to learn to manipulate the body and to communicate, all require effort. To learn language and to walk as a child are often painful and painstaking experiences.

These lessons are forgotten as we grow older, for gradually the hard-won skills become relatively effortless. We then move on to toilet training, eating with cutlery, schooling, career and so on. If we wish to learn anything at all it requires effort, so why wouldn't this apply in the case of love? Perhaps it does. Perhaps what has been discussed so far has nothing to do with love at all, and love remains an unknown quantity.

What does effort imply? Obviously, what we usually call effort or work has little to do with what we usually call love. On the whole, effort is the expenditure of energy in order to fulfil a need, and on the basic physical level this means food, clothing, housing and medicine.

We then move on to what we see as psychological or emotional needs and apply a certain amount of physical effort to fulfil these, but on the whole expect that they should come under the category of recreation, or rewards for the energy expended in physical or mental work.

If we look at what effort or work implies, we find that it is, in some ways, a repetition of an action, and if we look closer we see that in repeating an action, the possibility for bringing awareness to it increases. If we repeat with a minimum of awareness we will eventually be able to continue the action simply by physical habit, but if the awareness is focussed on the action, there comes a moment when the awareness and the physical action come to a point of balance and the action becomes effortless. All skills and crafts are built on this principle.

Naturally, this cannot occur if we are not interested in the action we perform, and only do it out of coercion of one form or another. This means either punishment or reward, and it must be admitted that many people run their lives on this basis.

*   *   *

If it is awareness which brings work to a point where it is effortless, is it possible that awareness has something to do with love? Certainly awareness is based on interest, for if something excites our interest we are definitely aware of it. Is it then possible that interest is linked with love?

This might be worth testing, and it is pertinent to note that the word *interest* means in Latin, "it concerns, it is of importance", and derives from *inter* and *esse* meaning "to be between". This implies movement from one point to another, but it is also the position in which both points can still be referred to—a position of balance. If something is of concern or importance, it means that there is a movement towards it—a focussing on it—while at the same time being aware of our reactions to it.

One way of testing this would be to stop doing what we think we should, ought or have been told to do, or what we do simply because we know how to or have a gift for, and see what interests us. If we find that there is something which genuinely concerns us, we could try doing that, which entails making a conscious decision about it and moving towards it.

This means that we have a good chance of developing a high degree of awareness in what we are doing. It doesn't necessarily mean that our lives will become suddenly and magically transformed or that they will suddenly become effortless, but there is the possibility that what we do will gradually become effortless as the physical effort is taken over more and more by the awareness.

This raises the question of vocation, for vocation is the willingness to expend effort where we are concerned and interested. It is often said that vocation is doing what we love, and so we wait for what we love to magically show up in order that we might be carried away by it and do it.

Perhaps the beginning of questioning what is meant by love is to give up all preconceived ideas and assumptions about it and be willing to base our work and the fulfilling of our physical needs on the risk of committing ourselves to what interests and concerns us.

This requires a complete re-evaluation of priorities, for we usually work at what the market dictates in order to get ahead, be secure, and so on. There is a definite risk in putting the effort into what interests us, as there is no guarantee of any success or reward. However, if we are interested and concerned, external reward is not a major priority, and it is this realisation which marks the dividing line between adulthood and childhood—the point of maturity.

*   *   *

The issues of awareness, interest and vocation bring into question the second assumption about love, namely that it is something we "fall into". Falling into something automatically implies lack of awareness, for to fall in means not seeing, or choosing not to see, what was there in the first place. It also implies not having a choice, and it certainly implies that no decision was made.

Therefore, the issue could not have been of any concern or importance, for if it were it would have been seen and then it would have been impossible to fall into. Something which is seen can either be walked around, or into, or we can lower ourselves into it or jump in, but it is impossible to fall in.

This assumption then asserts that love is based on a lack of awareness and all that implies, but most people would certainly deny that they have no concern for those they love. However, if they "fall in" love, it means just that.

And so we come to a point of contradiction—or else a deliberate untruth. Perhaps it means that a choice was made *not* to see what really was there, but to hope that the situation would fulfill what was perceived as a need. Then the interest or concern was directed towards fulfilling a perceived need and was not directed towards the situation or the person involved.

Certainly this concurs with the first assumption: that love is something which has to be obtained from someone else. Therefore, the awareness is not directed towards the other person, but is focussed on whether they are providing the need for whatever love is perceived to be. Love then, under these conditions, is not an act of concern, interest or awareness for others, but is a need.

What is this need? Is it to be fed? When we were infants this was a real need, but as adults is it genuinely so? We certainly need to eat, but do we really need to lie down and have someone pour food into our mouths? Obviously not—we are quite capable of feeding ourselves.

Of course this does not necessarily mean that some don't want to lie down and be fed. Therefore, a very clear distinction must be made between what is a real need and what we want. If love is perceived as being looked after and being fed by others in adulthood, this is not a need but a want.

It would then be more correct to define love under these conditions as a state of wanting, and it is interesting to remember that wanting also means lacking. It must also be seen whether what we want has any connection with reality. This will be discussed later.

*   *   *

Is there a genuine need which could be perceived as having something to do with love? Returning to the mother and the infant, let us examine the feelings of fulfilment and contentment which follow being fed. Is it this which is meant by love? Are these real needs?

In infancy, this would arise from having a full stomach and being held by our mother. As adults, having full stomachs does not necessarily mean that we feel fulfilled or contented. Being held might mean so—it all depends on who is holding us.

This means that if we perceive our fulfilment as being dependent on being held by someone else, we are obliged to make sure that someone else is there to do it, and to make sure that they do it when required and in the fashion required.

We find, however, that if they do it too often or not enough, and if they hold on too long, it ceases to be fulfilling and becomes uncomfortable. Hence, what should be a pleasant situation becomes painful. This follows for all pleasurable situations; they always stop, and if they go on too long they become painful. Naturally, this also applies to full stomachs.

It might have been noticed, too, that establishing and maintaining a situation where the right person is holding us at the right time (provided also that we are capable of knowing when the right time is), would require a considerable amount of effort. This goes against the third assumption about love. The effort in this case is put into making sure that someone is there, that they are there all the time, that they respond when required, that they stop when we've had enough and that they don't make uncomfortable demands upon us.

We might be willing to pay them to do it—for example, some forms of marriage, prostitution, and servants—but if not, we must be prepared to face the fact that anyone who agrees to these conditions is probably demanding the same thing themselves. Usually this fact is not faced and the demands on both sides are covert. If they remain so, the relationship continues. Once the demands become overt, the relationship often breaks down—which entails starting all over again. It is beginning to look as though no matter how we perceive love, it requires effort.

*   *   *

Is fulfilment a genuine need? As adults, our survival is certainly not dependent on being held, so it appears this again comes under the category of wanting and is not a need. On the other hand, life without fulfilment, contentment or happiness is certainly an intolerable situation, even though it is possible to survive physically without them. So it appears that there could be a case for establishing these as emotional and psychological needs. If this is so, the question then arises as to how to meet them.

Once the obvious physical needs are met, we are then faced with the question of how we feel. We tend to think that our feelings are dependent on how these physical needs are met, for example, food. That is, we confuse the way we feel with the way in which our physical needs are met: "If only the food had been cooked in this way instead of that, I would feel much better". We do not see that there is a clear distinction between physical needs and feelings. Once the need is met, how we feel depends much more on our state of mind than on how the need was met.

It has been seen that in infancy, how we feel is totally dependent on whether our mothers feed and clothe us or not, and how they hold us. In adulthood, this is not the case. We are perfectly capable of fulfilling these needs ourselves, for we have the freedom and the capacity to do so. Our dialogues can then cease to be based on the power struggles resulting from assumed states of dependency, and become balanced and mutual.

*   *   *

It would seem that the three assumptions about love are a state of confusion over remembered experiences of childhood, for they are an attempt to repeat in one way or another what we actually experienced as infants. This situation becomes even more confused when these experiences were unhealthy in some way.

For example, our mothers might have been emotionally upset, or in an extremely stressful situation, or subject to violence or addicted to a drug of some kind. These emotions and the accompanying physical odours would then have been an integral part of our feeding experience and we would automatically have identified them with love and so attempt to repeat them.

We do not appear to notice that these experiences no longer apply, and so trying to repeat them requires an effort of which we are unaware. Our focus is on the supposed need, and so the effort goes into not seeing what the situation actually is or who the other person with whom we are dialoguing is. We are simply trying to manipulate the situation or person in an attempt to fulfill this supposed need. As the need is no longer a reality, the whole dialogue with the situation or person is ultimately doomed.

This is what unhealthy desire or craving is—a memory of past experience which we cling to and project on to present situations where it has no relevance. This creates a great deal of conflict because of course the desire is insatiable, as it has no ground in reality and therefore can never be fulfilled.

A state of wanting or desire, therefore, is what is commonly meant by love. Desire is usually what is perceived as a psychological need. All unhealthy desire, then, stems from a refusal to admit that we are no longer infants and are quite capable of supplying our own physical needs.

If we give way to this form of desire, we are simply attempting to seduce others into believing that we are children and that therefore we need to be looked after. As has been pointed out, this cannot lead to anything but dissatisfaction.

We have seen that no matter which way we play it, effort is required. We can either put effort into manipulating people and situations to fulfil our insatiable cravings, or we can put it into being aware of the situations we are in and the people we are dialoguing with. In the latter case, we are prepared to move our awareness away from our own supposed needs or wants, and place it in our environment.

This is the dividing line between childhood and adulthood—the moment of maturity—for we are prepared to invest our energies in what surrounds us, without seeking the gratification of our wants. This movement of awareness away from memories, fantasies and wants, to what actually is around us, is the gift of interest which we give to others. Vocation is the first step in this direction.

We are then in a position to make a clear distinction between physical needs and feelings, and not confuse the two. We are capable of seeing clearly the reality we are dialoguing with, and we do not have our energies being drained off into maintaining dialogues of unawareness where we are committed to not seeing.

Therefore, we have the awareness, energy and interest to direct our questioning to our feelings, and consider what it means to be fulfilled. We will find that we are dealing with a level of reality which is much more subtle than physical feeding. Of course, we do not have the possibility of considering fulfilment until the physical needs are met, but they alone will not satisfy the feelings.

*   *   *

Feelings are something within ourselves and require a completely different orientation of perception. It is necessary to cease looking outside ourselves for their fulfilment. Instead, we need to soften and dissolve the hard, callous and sentimental attitudes we have towards ourselves and be prepared to open to the very fine, subtle sensations within the body. It is possible, once our awareness is brought to bear on them, to cultivate these fine sensations so that they open and pervade our entire body.

We will then discover that every action we perform, everything we say, every interaction we take part in and everything we think, sets off a whole range of feelings. When we breathe, it is possible to feel the breath enter and permeate our entire body. We can become aware of the very fine internal sensations which respond to each sense stimulus.

As this aspect of our lives is developed, we find that every resonance within us can be brought to full awareness, and thus there is a very real connection between how we feel and what is happening around us. We become aware of the feeling that every breath nourishes our bodies, as do sights, sounds, tastes, odours and contacts with the skin; that in fact we are being supported and held in an environment that is constantly feeding us on a very subtle level. In this sense the earth is also our mother.

As this awareness grows and develops, we come to discover fulfilment, for there is not one single moment when we are not, in actuality, being fed or supported in one way or another. Our culture, friends, colleagues, those we don't even know who supply all the goods and services we take for granted, and even those we see as our enemies, are feeding us. This of course entails giving up the fixed ideas of how we think we want to be fed and supported, and being prepared to invest our interest and awareness in how it is actually happening.

Love then is not, as is usually supposed, a desire to repeat remembered personal experiences. It is a feeling within us which comes from opening ourselves to the inner sensations of our bodies as they respond to the life and the world around them. It is a communication with, a movement of genuine interest and awareness towards, our partners and friends, our community, our environment and the world. This resonates throughout our whole body, at a very fine and subtle level, so that no part of us is held in reserve or left out of the communication.

It is total. It depends on making the move towards, and of committing ourselves to, our environment—the places and people with whom we are associated. When this communication is total, when nothing is left out, there can be no sense of emptiness, alienation or unfulfilment.

We are then filled with what surrounds us and are able to embrace it with our interest and awareness. There is no separation between what we perceive and the perception itself—we are our environment and it is us.

When the illusion of separation and its accompanying pain of alienation dissolve, there is fulfilment, joy and love.

Living without awareness
is dreaming.

Trade in memories and habit-patterns
for clear awareness.

Accept what no-one else wants and
transform it by loving it.

CHAPTER **5** | *Calm and concentration—*
balancing body and mind

When the body and emotions
are calm, the mind is naturally
concentrated, because it is
totally absorbed. The state
of absorption gives a feeling
of rapture—a cool, blissful
ecstasy—far beyond the feelings
derived from physical pleasure.

The body of meditation work takes the mind beyond questions and answers to direct experience. Looking for an answer only hinders the unfolding of direct experience, for it presupposes the outcome of what is being done. In this preoccupied state, it is not possible to see what is actually happening.

Wanting results is therefore the main hindrance to seeing clearly. This leads to dissatisfaction, anger, lack of interest, lethargy and boredom as the desired results are not forthcoming. Then restlessness and worry set in as the attempt is made to manufacture results. Finally indecision and self-doubt take over the mind as the feeling sets in that it is impossible to meditate with any success and develop calm and concentration.

All of this is the outcome of looking for predetermined results, and so the body of meditation work is a way of developing and deepening calm so that the mind can open to the immediate present, no matter how trivial what is happening might appear to be. In fact, the focus is often especially on those things which we think are not important, for one of the major ways of protecting preconceptions and fixed ideas is to dismiss as trivial what does not fit in with them.

In being able to sustain the state of question, the way is prepared for developing mental tranquillity and insight. The foundation practices can be done in daily life along with our ordinary activities, and a good deal of the practice of developing calm can be done in this way also.

Everyday life also provides plenty of opportunities for developing awareness. By using meditation to calm and balance the mind and emotions through bringing them to the point where they are momentarily still, it is possible to detach the mind from the habitual and powerful emotions which affect everyone's life. It is then possible to see options which would not normally be seen. This gives the opportunity to make decisions with awareness in situations where habitual emotions would make this impossible to do.

All meditation work is for opening and deepening awareness, and this—the body of meditation practice—is a simple, efficient yet profound way of doing this. The practice itself is divided into two parts: the development of mental tranquillity or absorbed concentration, and the development of insight or wisdom.

Mental tranquillity

There are six categories of meditation for the development of mental tranquillity or one-pointed concentration: the state of complete absorption of mind. They have evolved to suit the different needs of different people, and so it is not necessary to work through all of them. If there is one which suits you, then that is the one to take and cultivate, because keeping the work as simple as possible is the most effective way for it to unfold.

Of course, if you wish to explore a wide range, by all means do so for the essence of these practices is to open to new experience or, more accurately, to new and wider ranges of perception. This constitutes part of the dialogue with a teacher— ascertaining what suits the needs of the individual.

Breathing

Breathing meditation is the simplest, most straightforward of all meditation practices, and the one which will carry the mind right through to insight. This is the practice of maintaining awareness of the breath either at the tip of the nose, or at the chest or belly. There are two ways of doing breathing meditation—either through counting the individual breaths (usually from one to ten), or just through spontaneous awareness of the breath. The latter is the best preparation for insight.

Visualisation

This is the study of the creation and dissolution of experiences in the mind. It could be called creative imagination. Visualisation is an exploration of the infinite variety of shapes, colours, images and patterns created by the mind. The practice is designed for becoming aware of the fact that our minds contain all the varieties and potentialities of all behaviour, from the wildest and most energetic to the most sublime and serene, and that what we visualise can help shape our own behaviour and experience.

The Tibetan tradition is particularly rich in visualisation practices which can be adapted for Western use. They are invariably done in conjunction with mantra. This category also includes taking visual external objects for meditation, such as colours, light and natural objects.

Mantra

Mantra is the practice of meditating upon sounds as word-symbols. There are three kinds:

- Pure sound: sound or seed syllables, without any particular meaning, which resonate with specific areas of the body, thereby deepening awareness of directly focussed feelings and experiences. Examples of these are the syllables OM, AH and HUM.

- Sound and form: combinations of seed syllables with words, co-ordinated with particular visualisations. An example of this is the mantra used with the washing meditation: OM VAJRA SATTVA HUM.

Another example of this is the most famous Tibetan mantra of all, the mantra of compassion: OM MANI PADME HUM, where MANI means "jewel", symbolising the crystal clear quality of mind, the depth of our being, and PADME means "lotus", or any kind of flower which, in growing from a seed in the ground and then unfolding into full life, symbolises the body. The fact that our own lives and bodies are an embodiment of the matrix of consciousness—that vibrant, luminous, spacious quality of mind—is the essence of compassion. Keeping the mind and body connected and in a balanced state is the essence of any act of compassion.

- Reflective mantras which embody philosophical ideas for contemplation.

This category also includes meditations on natural sounds.

Bodily energies

The practice of meditating on the energies of the body includes meditating on the points where energies focus, traditionally referred to as *chakras*. Chakra literally means "wheel", and so takes on the meaning of an energy centre which radiates from a core. They are often presented as being fixed shapes and colours, and associated with particular organs, but this is misleading. A more accurate perception is of fields and fluxing of energy. These can either be seen as colours which float in the mind and change according to the way the states of mind and emotions change, or felt as sensations in particular parts of the body.

There is a group of six tantric yogas in the Tibetan tradition called the Six Yogas of Naropa through which this practice can be developed to a high degree. These include yogas for centring the energies of the body; for working with dreams; for working with inner light; and for becoming aware of how formations come into being and pass away.

Movement

There are a number of ways of developing calm and concentration through movement; perhaps the best known are yoga and Tai Chi. In the Tibetan tradition there is a body of exercises known as Kum Nye, which are used to attain a deeply relaxed state of body and mind.

Contemplation

These meditations are directed to the emotions. They focus on qualities which give rise to inspiration, and so open the way for cultivating these qualities in the life. Inspirational meditations are based in the heart and draw us into a wider and deeper view of life. They are used for consciously developing the qualities of love, respect, devotion, awe, and so on—qualities which allow us to feel and value our lives and the lives of all others. Four examples of these are the formal meditations on all-embracing kindness, compassion, joy, and the state of complete balance and equanimity—a sense of deep inner peace.

Developing mental tranquillity is the way of opening to new experience: to new, more embracing forms of perception. This gives rise to inspiration because inspiration itself is the feeling of opened perception. Insight is the co-ordination, the referencing of new experience, so that it can be assimilated.

The state of absorption

When the body and emotions are calm, the mind is naturally concentrated, because it is totally absorbed. The state of absorption gives a feeling of rapture—a cool, blissful ecstasy—far beyond the feelings derived from physical pleasure.

There are two types of absorption:

- the absorption of ecstasy or joy, which once attained will propel the mind to the other type of absorption;

- the absorption of direct experience or direct knowing which will lead to insight.

Concentration itself is a state of calm, and there are six factors which arise when this is established:

- a focussing of the mind as it ceases to be distracted;

- an ability for the mind to rest gently on the object taken for meditation, scanning and exploring it;

- a pleasurable interest, which can extend right through to complete ecstasy;

- a state of happiness or satisfaction as the mind correlates and digests the information given;

- the bringing of the mind to complete one-pointedness;

- a state of resolution, experienced as balance or equanimity.

There are three similes used to describe the stages of settling the mind, for in the beginning it can be quite a shock to discover the amount of mental traffic which passes through it. Often people think meditation has caused a sudden influx of thoughts; however, this is only seeing for the first time just how much is going on in the mind.

- The first stage is compared with a steep mountain waterfall, as the rush of thoughts and images passing through the mind enters awareness.

- The second is compared with a large, gentle, steadily flowing river, as the traffic thins out and thoughts and images settle of their own accord.

- The third is described as being like the river flowing into the sea, for at this stage all conceptualisation is released completely and the mind settles into a blissful state of equipoise.

There is no need to push or try to force thoughts and images to disappear. They will dissolve quite naturally of their own accord, as the mind is gently held on the object of meditation.

Because the mind and energies of the body are inseparable, it is essential to develop the ability to contain the energies in order for the mind to become settled. Unfortunately, a great deal of superstition and guilt have grown up around the question of sexuality within both the Western and Eastern meditation traditions. However, the situation is very straightforward.

Naturally when meditating, it is impossible for the mind to become calm and develop concentration if we are obsessively thinking of someone else, or if we are stroking someone's thigh and having our ears nibbled. Therefore it is important to learn to contain our energies, which means to be self-contained. A healthy basis on which this can be done is to cultivate relaxed, healthy relationships with others. In both friendships and sexual relations this means relationships which embody healthy feeling qualities: true caring, respect, consideration, sympathy and independence.

Promiscuity, like lasciviousness, enforced celibacy and a puritanical attitude to sexuality, are all ways of repressing feelings, and so can only lead to agitation and anxiety. They are therefore not conducive to developing calm. Too often so-called celibacy is used as a licence to indulge the will by attempting to dominate others.

When the energies of the body are balanced we naturally become self-contained, and so are in an effortlessly blissful state. *Contained* and *contented* come from the same root, meaning in Latin "to hold together"; it is when we have the ability to hold our energies together that we become contented, and have a real choice about what we do with our life energies.

The four meditation postures

As was outlined in chapter 3, a comfortable, stable, alert posture is also necessary for the cultivation of calm. Meditation can be done while sitting, walking, standing or lying down. Each of these postures can be used either formally or informally.

The formal postures are:

- For sitting, either use a straight-backed padded chair (or armchair) or a fairly high cushion or meditation stool, so that the spine is comfortably erect with the chin slightly tucked in to open the back of the neck. The hands are either rested on the thighs, or together in the lap. The belly is relaxed and the eyes are softened, either closed or half-opened. The jaw, tongue and shoulders are also relaxed.

(This posture was outlined in detail in chapter 3.)

- For walking, hold the hands, right in left, either in front or behind, letting the arms hang naturally. Walk slowly, with small steps, in a straight line for about 17 paces or so (depending on the length of the path or room), then turn slowly and walk back. Repeat this for the duration of the session.

- For standing, stand with the back against a wall, with the hands held in front as for walking.

• For lying down, either lie on the back with the arms at the sides, hands open, or lie on the right side with the right hand underneath the face, the legs together with the knees slightly bent and the left arm down the left side of the body.

In the beginning, short, frequent sessions are the best way to develop mental tranquillity. Meditating is very pleasant and there is nothing to be achieved through forcing and trying to make the sessions long and therefore uncomfortable and unpleasant. The mind will not settle under these conditions, so it is fruitless to continue once having become tired.

While fresh, and while the interest is there, meditating will be pleasant and the habit will build up naturally. Therefore, breaking the session while the mind is still clear, and taking a rest, will eliminate the possibility of becoming bored. Meditating will then remain enjoyable and interesting.

Eventually, once concentration has been developed, it is possible to hold the mind still without focussing on any object at all. To put it more precisely, we will be able simply to take space as the object of meditation. It is at this stage that the work will turn naturally to insight.

The signs of mental tranquillity

When the mind is settled and quiet thoughts still come and go; however, they do not get stuck. Any thought, image or sensation flows straight through the mind without getting caught. The mind is clear like a mirror and reflects what happens without getting involved with it in any way. At this stage it does not matter what kind of thoughts or images come along, there is no reaction to them at all, and the mind can remain stable, alert and clear.

Calm and concentration are dependent on each other. Because the mind focuses on a meditation object it is not distracted by whatever else passes through and so rests calmly in that one place. If we do get drawn into a passing thought or sensation, the meditation object provides an anchor to which we can return and so hold the mind steady.

It is important to be able to recognise when we are holding the mind too loosely or too tightly on the object. If our focus is too loose we will find that we tend to become dull or dazed as our mind drifts off and starts to wander aimlessly. When this happens we will find the body has started to slump and so a good way to tighten concentration is to check the posture. Check too that the room is fresh and airy and hasn't become too warm and stuffy. It is useful to know that lifting the focus of the eyes slightly also sharpens concentration.

If the focus is too tight we will be agitated and will probably find that we are tense, perhaps trying too hard, and that our mind is jumping around so much that it cannot settle in one place. In this state we can find that our eyes are staring, even if they are closed, and so softening and slightly lowering their focus can help. However, more often than not, once agitation sets in the best thing to do is to break the meditation session for a while and do some physical exercise.

Being calm and concentrated is an extremely pleasant state, and there are three qualities which always arise once the mind settles. These are the three signs of mental tranquillity. They are traditionally called *bliss, clarity* and *non-conceptuality*.

Bliss refers to the body—the feeling of deep relaxation and peace which comes as tight muscles and knots in the energies of the body loosen. At the same time the body is tingling with energy; a vital, vibrant feeling which permeates the whole body.

Clarity refers to the mind which is clear like a mirror; alert and aware, clinging to nothing but simply reflecting whatever passes through.

Non-conceptuality means that the mind is not thinking about

whatever sensations are presented to it. Whatever comes to the mind is perceived without any thought, so that no concepts are formed around what is experienced or seen. This gives a feeling of spaciousness as the mind rests in the open space free from thought.

These three qualities are an integral part of mental tranquillity, and so give a clear sign that it has been established. Once they are present, maintaining calm and concentration becomes effortless, and meditating flows smoothly of its own accord.

CHAPTER **6** | *Meditations for developing calm and concentration*

Before meditating formally it is a good idea to do some exercises to loosen the body, to let go of the tension which builds up during everyday life. Initially, many of the difficulties people have when beginning to meditate come from the physical tension they are holding in their bodies.

The six kinds of calming meditation

Once you are seated, and before beginning a formal meditation, rock gently from side to side, allowing the movement to become smaller and smaller until your body finds its own balance point.

Exhale fully and take a deep breath into your abdomen. Then exhale slowly. This will help relax your body. Now you are ready to begin a formal meditation, and there are six categories to choose from.

Breathing

There are two kinds of breathing meditation—one is spontaneous and involves simply being aware of the breath as it moves through the nostrils, and the other is controlled. There are a wide range of controlled breathing meditations, including the pranayama exercises of yoga and the practices of Tantra.

- The simplest meditation of all is to watch or feel your breath at the nostrils. Place your awareness at the tip of your nose and observe the breath entering and leaving your body. While doing this, register each in-breath and out-breath in the mind by thinking "breathing in", "breathing out".

- An alternative form of breathing meditation is to count each breath. An in-and out-breath counts as one breath; these are counted from one to ten, with the count at the end of the out-breath. The process is repeated for the duration of the session.

- A simple form of controlled breathing meditation is to breathe in deeply, right down to your belly; hold the breath for a while, as long as is comfortable, and then breathe out slowly.

Vase breathing

The traditional meditation called *vase breathing* is a major practice in the yoga-tantras.

- Expel the air from your body and then take a long, deep breath into the pit of your stomach. Use your abdominal muscles to gently push the breath down below the navel so that your abdomen hangs out like a pot or a vase. Then slightly tighten the muscles around your anus. Hold this breath for as long as you can. Then raise your head slightly and release the air as slowly as possible.

This exercise works best if you keep it gentle, so don't force it, and do it for a maximum of six breaths in any one session.

Visualisation

A very effective meditation is to visualise light moving through your body.

- Visualise a large sphere of peach-coloured light above your head. From this sphere, a stream of light flows into the top of your head and through your body, gradually filling it with peach-coloured light. Feel the light penetrating every part of your body. Dissolve the visualisation by bringing all the light to your heart centre, at the centre of your chest, where it shrinks to a pinpoint and disappears.

Mind and body washing

This meditation is a variation on the washing meditation given in chapter 4.

- Visualise a misty shower of sun-filled rain washing over and through your body. Let this sun-filled rain soak through the top of your head and wash through all your bones, nervous system, your blood system, organs and muscles, allowing the rain to leave your body through your fingers and toes. It doesn't have to be exact; just imagining this is enough. To complete the meditation, allow the rain to turn to light then bring it to your heart centre, where it shrinks to a pinpoint of light and disappears.

Meditating on colour

For this meditation you need to create a disc of colour—either colour in a piece of white cardboard or glue coloured paper onto cardboard, about 20 to 30 centimetres in diameter. The colours traditionally used are deep blue, yellow, red, white and green.

- Place the disc about a metre in front of you, lower than your eyes, so that you are looking slightly downwards. Close your eyes, then open them about half-way to soften and relax them and allow your mind to rest gently on the colour to absorb it. Then close your eyes and see if you can still see the colour by visualising it.

Meditating on visual objects

To meditate on visual objects, use a stone, flower, crystal or any other object which interests you.

- Close your eyes, then open them about half-way to soften and relax them and allow your mind to rest gently on the visual object.

Informal meditation

An informal way to use visualisation is to meditate on reflected light when you are outside.

- Let your eyes focus gently on the light on the leaves of trees or the reflected light on water. You can allow your mind to rest in the light so that your awareness dissolves into the light.

Mantra

Mantra simply means meditating on sound. This can be done by imagining the sounds in your mind or by listening to sounds around you.

Seed syllables

Meditating on the syllables OM AH HUM (pronounced HOONG) is a simple and useful mantra to use.

- Say or sing out loud OM AH HUM, or imagine the sound in your mind.

Mantras

Two very useful mantras are HAMSA and ARAHAM.

- To meditate using the mantra HAMSA, which can be translated approximately as "I am complete", first say the HAM (pronounced HUM), and then let the SA (pronounced SAR) come out slowly like a sigh. You can also say this mantra silently in your mind, saying the HAM on the in-breath and the SA on the out-breath.

• The mantra ARAHAM can be loosely translated as "freedom". It is pronounced AH RAH HUNG, and while repeating it out loud or silently in your mind, you can visualise a golden light through your body or a large bell tolling.

Meditating on sound

A good way to begin every meditation is to meditate on all the sounds around you, allowing them into your meditation no matter what they are.

• Listen around you in every direction, letting all the sounds in the room, in the building, and outside, to enter your mind and body. Listen out as far as you can. You will find that you can allow your awareness to just rest in the sensation of sound.

Listening to music is another effective way to meditate on sound.

• Once you have set yourself up for meditating, turn on the music and allow your mind to focus on it in the same way you meditate on the sounds around you. As you listen, your mind will become increasingly absorbed in the music and you may feel your body resonating to the sound—as if you are feeling the music inside your body.

Informal meditation

An informal way to meditate on sound is to become aware of the sounds around you while walking, letting them all into your awareness. This is particularly beautiful if you are walking along a beach listening to the sounds of the sea, or in a park or the country where you can hear birds and other sounds of nature around you.

Bodily energies

There are a number of different ways to meditate on bodily energies.

Breathing

- Begin with the simple breathing meditation, becoming aware of your breathing at the nostrils. Then become aware of your chest rising and falling as you breathe, and the gentle movement of your stomach. Slightly slow down the in-breath and follow it into the heart centre at the centre of your chest. Then, on the out-breath, imagine the breath spreading through your entire body and leaving through the skin.

Breathing—variation

A variation is to follow the in-breath to the pit of the stomach, then imagine the out-breath spreading through your entire body and leaving through the skin.

One of these variations will probably feel more comfortable. If so, keep that as your preferred option.

Visualisation

The visualisation used with the practice of prostrations can be used as a meditation on its own.

- Visualise a white light at the forehead and say, either out loud or silently, the syllable OM. Then visualise a red light at the throat while saying the syllable AH. And finally visualise a deep blue light at the heart centre, at the centre of the chest, while saying the syllable HUM (pronounced HOONG).

Body scan

Scanning through the body in sections, while watching all the sensations at those particular areas, is a form of meditating on the energies of the body. You can become aware of the variations in sensation at the different energy centres of the body.

• Start at the top of the head and forehead, noticing all the sensations there, whether pleasant, painful or neutral. Feel the tingling or pressure in the head. Then move to the face and lower part of the head. Soften the eyes and loosen the jaw. Then move to the throat and neck, shoulders, arms, hands and fingers.
Move to the chest and upper back. Feel the lungs expand and contract and the movement of your ribs and diaphragm as you breathe. Move to the abdomen and lower back and notice all the sensations there, feeling the organs moving as you breathe.
And finally notice all the sensations in the hips, legs feet and toes. Feel or imagine the breath dropping through your body. Now let your mind rest at any place in your body. Watch and feel the breath moving in that place and notice any sensations there.

Movement

Rocking from side to side

This meditation is a particularly good one to use each time you sit down to meditate.

• Rock your torso gently from side to side, allowing the movement to get smaller and smaller, rather like a pendulum swinging, until your body finds its own balance point. Then do the same with your head and neck, letting them rock gently from side to side, allowing the movement to become smaller and smaller, until it too finds its own balance point.

Lowering shoulders

This movement meditation focuses on using your arms to lower your shoulders as slowly as possible.

- Place your hands on your thighs while sitting down. Then use your arms to push your shoulders up as high as possible and hold the stretch for a short time. Then very slowly bring your shoulders back down, keeping your awareness in the sensations of the movement. When you think you have finished, allow your shoulders to keep moving down until it is no longer possible to move them.

Flying

This movement meditation focuses on the sensations in your arms as you slowly raise them in an arc above your head.

- Stand with your feet slightly apart and your eyes either half-open or closed and let your arms hang loosely at your sides. Then bring your arms up by slowly lifting them away from the sides of your body in a curve until your hands meet over your head. Allow the hands to meet and have a little stretch. Then bring them down, following the same curve, just as slowly, keeping your awareness in the sensations of the movement.

You may wish to do this movement just once, or to extend the meditation, repeat the movement two more times.

Contemplation

Kindness

You can use contemplation to create feelings of kindness and acceptance towards yourself. As you repeat these phrases you may find these warm feelings growing through your whole body.

Say out loud or silently in your mind:

> May I be filled with kindness.
>
> May I be well.

May I be peaceful and at ease.

May I be happy.

Visualisation—kindness towards yourself

In this meditation, contemplating kindness is linked with a visualisation.

- Imagine a deep red rose in the heart centre, from which a soft light (either a soft pink or simply a white light) spreads through your whole body. With this light come feelings of kindness, warmth, acceptance and understanding which flow to every part of your body, to your thoughts, memories and emotions, and to your whole life.

Visualisation—kindness towards others

You can also extend this meditation to others.

- Imagine in front of you someone you love and embrace them in this light. Then imagine someone you wouldn't normally take any notice of—someone who doesn't seem very important to you or whom you have met just casually. Embrace them with this light of kindness. Finally, bring to mind someone you are afraid of, or who has caused you pain, and embrace them too with this light filled with kindness and understanding.

  Then let go of these images and bring the light back into your own body. Finish the meditation by allowing the light to return to the rose in your heart, then let the rose close to form a bud and get smaller until it becomes a pinpoint of light, and allow it to disappear. Let your mind rest with the feeling that has been generated in your body.

Walking meditation

There are a number of ways to meditate while walking.

Formal walking meditations

Set up the formal posture for walking meditation.

- Hold the hands, right in left, either in front or behind, letting the arms hang naturally. Walk slowly, with small steps, in a straight line for about 17 paces or so (depending on the length of the path or room), then turn slowly and walk back. Repeat this for the duration of the session.

The most detailed way of doing walking meditation is to become aware of the movement of your feet.

- Keep your mind on the three parts of each step by saying in your mind, "Lifting, moving, placing" as you move each foot.

You can also concentrate on the breath while walking by watching or feeling the breath moving in and out of your body.

- Either watch or feel the breath moving in and out of your nostrils, or feel the physical movement of your chest or stomach rising and falling. Choose whichever way is more comfortable for you. Keep your mind with the breath by saying in the mind: "Breathing in, breathing out" with each breath.

- A variation on this is to keep your breath in time with each step by discovering how many breaths you take for each step. For example, you might find that you breathe in for two steps and out for three steps. Often the out-breath is a little longer than the in-breath.

Informal walking meditations

Informal walking meditation can be done any time you go for a walk.

- Simply become aware of the movement of your body as you walk.

- As you walk, open your senses to the sounds around you; to the colours and the reflected light on leaves and water; to the feel of the air on your skin; and to the smells in the air.

• Feel the contact of your feet with the earth and cultivate a feeling of embracing the earth with your feet.

To complete this section, a reminder from chapter 5. All the different kinds of meditations have evolved to suit the needs of different people, so it is unnecessary to work through all of them. If there is one which suits you, then cultivate that, because keeping the work as simple as possible is the most effective way for it to unfold.

Thought is not the cause of
conflict and suffering—it is
the attachment to thought.
Or to anything.

As nothing lasts, there is
nothing to worry about.

Life is not nice; having to
be nice is suffering.

CHAPTER 7

Clear and open—beyond answers

Instead of looking for answers about the way the human mind and consciousness work and how this affects our experience of the world, Insight meditation provides the way to actually see and experience our mind and consciousness directly.

Once mental tranquillity is established, awareness stabilises. The calm then becomes alert and attentive. When the mind is calm and open, it can be brought to a state of intensity which is impossible to sustain under ordinary conditions. With this balanced intensity the opportunity to examine closely the nature of the mind itself arises.

This is the function of penetrative Insight meditation, for with insight we can cut through all preconceptions and habit patterns, freeing ourselves from them totally, and come to see correlations, options and alternatives which normally would be inconceivable.

Insight meditation is the practice of moving beyond knowledge based on ideas to knowledge based on direct experience. Instead of looking for answers about the way the human mind and consciousness work and how this affects our experience of the world, Insight meditation provides the way to actually see and experience our mind and consciousness directly. From there it is possible to see thoughts and the process of thinking—how thoughts come and go in the mind. Then we can see the relationship between the mind and the world around us, and how the way our mind works affects the way we experience the world.

Penetrative Insight meditation is done by waking up the calm. What this means is that once calm and concentration is established, the mind can rest effortlessly in one place—it is not distracted, restless, agitated, or dull. Thoughts and emotions become quiet and still and the body is relaxed, so that the mind and body reach a state of balance or equilibrium. In this state it is then possible to sharpen the mind by consciously using thought to give definition to this very open, calm and relaxed state. This can be done by holding a question like, "Where is the mind?" or "What does the mind look like?"

Insight meditation usually needs to be done under formal conditions where outer distractions and preoccupations are reduced to a minimum. In reducing sense stimulation, simplifying and slowing down your life under full-time meditation conditions, the focus of your awareness will eventually turn of its own accord from the world of phenomena, both physical and mental, to the essence of mind itself. This will then be established as a realisation in your life: not as an answer, speculation or a concept, but as a real, direct experience. As everything we are and experience appears to us as a function of the mind, that is, as a perception of one sort or another, we will then know directly the seat of all perception.

* * *

The practice of penetrative insight is pure observation; just watching without censoring or attempting to change anything: seeing the mind as it is. It involves observing the mind while it is still, and observing the thoughts and images as they flow through. As was pointed out earlier, meditating on the natural, spontaneous flow of the breath is one meditation which will bring us to, and sustain us through the work of insight.

Penetrative insight involves watching the body, feelings and sensations, the states or qualities of the mind, and the objects the mind takes, that is, the thoughts and images. Observing the breath and its different rates (quick, slow, shallow, deep, and so on) is a way of focussing awareness on the body.

This will lead to becoming aware of the sensations associated with the different rates of breath, whether pleasant, painful or neutral. We will notice whether these sensations have a focal point in any particular part of the body.

As we are able to observe on more subtle levels, the qualities of mind (distracted, concentrated, busy, dull, kind, and so on) and the emotions associated with these qualities will become apparent. We will also notice how our sensations, emotions and breath patterns are linked and whether any emotion we are feeling has its focal point in a part of the body.

Then we will be able to watch, without distraction, the thoughts and images of the mind as they arise and dissolve. Seeing what arises, clearly and directly, no matter whether it is terrifying or exquisitely beautiful—just calmly observing without being moved at all—is the essence of Insight meditation.

One of the fundamental prerequisites for insight work is complete honesty, both with ourselves and with a teacher. No matter how strange or trivial what was seen might appear, that is what was seen, and it is only on the basis of direct simplicity that Insight meditation can be fruitful. As pointed out earlier, it is quite possible for insight to arise, and to see the nature of the mind, and not recognise it. One of the main functions of a teacher is to guide towards this recognition and to test it when it arises.

The four levels of insight

There are four ways of looking at the mind:

- when it is still and settled;

- when it is moving with thoughts and images;

- in relation to the body and appearances, that is, what appear to be external objects;

- when it is still together with when it is moving.

Once the four ways of looking at the mind are cultivated, these different aspects of the mind can be recognised. The act of recognition is a direct realisation or insight, and the four different ways of recognising the mind give a complete understanding of its nature.

These four realisations are four distinct moments of insight—they are definite experiences which arise individually and in order, often with a long period of time between them as each experience is integrated into everyday life. Each of these moments of insight can be tested to ensure there is complete understanding of what they show and what they mean.

Each insight reveals the nature of the mind from a particular point of view. The first insight is the first experience of actually seeing the mind when it is free from thoughts, concepts and images. It is calm and settled. This is the experience of "openness" or "emptiness" because the mind is "empty" of concepts and in this state is seen to be infinite and completely open.

What this reveals is that our identity is simply one concept among many, and that when there are no concepts in the mind there is no sense of "I" in the mind either. In the Buddhist tradition the first insight is called "entering the stream" because it is the first experience of directly seeing the mind without self-referencing. We see and feel ourselves as an integral part of our environment and of the universe as the sense of "separateness" which we take for granted completely dissolves. It is the first moment of realising what it is like to be free from being driven by wanting, anger and fear. This gives us the ability to see their cause.

The second insight shows that thoughts and concepts also have no solid core or basis, but, like clouds in the sky, are translucent, ephemeral and transparent. It shows too that thoughts are not created by us, but that they are a natural part of the mind. They arise and dissolve immediately. As we use thoughts to name everything we see in the world around us, this insight reveals what it is like to see everything without names, to see them as endlessly changing and fluxing rather than as fixed things.

The third insight is an insight into the relationship between our minds and bodies and between our minds and what appear to be external objects. It is seen that there is no separation between mind and body. As well, we discover that there is no separation between what we see and experience in the world and the thoughts and concepts we hold about them in our mind.

The fourth insight shows the relationship between the mind when it is still and when it is moving with thoughts. We see that the mind cannot be still and thinking at the same time. When it is still it is open, calm and free from concepts; when it is moving thoughts come and go of their own accord. However, no matter whether the mind is still or moving with thoughts, we see that it still has exactly the same quality of clarity and openness. The insight also shows that everything we are and experience is shaped totally by our perceptions. The open experience of our senses is shaped and determined by how we learn to name it.

In the Zen tradition, the four insights into the nature of mind are described as follows:

• Removing the subject:

the first insight where the mind is seen free from concepts and so is "empty" of thoughts, self-referencing and identity. "I" is therefore removed.

• Removing the object:

the second insight where objects in the world are seen free from the concepts which normally name them—they are perceived directly and so are removed as fixed objects.

• Removing both the subject and the object:

the third insight where both the mind and what it perceives are seen free from concepts and are seen to be inseparable. As both are empty and open, both are removed.

• Removing neither the subject nor the object:

the fourth insight where the objects we perceive are seen to be shaped and created by the concepts of the mind. Concepts and objects are seen and understood for what they are and so are not removed.

These are the four possible combinations of subject and object. This constitutes the dialogue which gives rise to self-consciousness, for self-consciousness only arises with an object.

*   *   *

It is possible to arrive at these insights through following all the stages of the mind as insight deepens. There are generally considered to be sixteen stages leading to insight, and these are developed through observing the breath and following the feelings, states of mind and the objects of mind. This particular practice focuses on the dialogue between mind and body.

The four insights are a direct experience of the nature of the mind or the operation of consciousness. This is the function of penetrative Insight meditation, for it is through this deep understanding that we are completely freed from being driven by what we do not comprehend. When the mind itself is seen and understood, there is complete freedom from conflicting emotions and states of confusion.

The first insight is the first direct seeing of the mind. This is what the Zen tradition calls *satori* and is the experience popularly known as enlightenment. The second liberates us from clinging to the objects of our wanting and fear. The third brings a state of total relief as the process of subject-object is completely seen through and as the foundation for our clinging, and the fear which accompanies it, are seen to be illusory. The fourth brings clear seeing and frees the mind from emotional conflict and confusion, as normal consciousness is directly experienced. Conceptualisation—the process of mental construction—and our sense experience are seen to be two different processes. Seeing is simply seeing, completely free from preconceptions.

*   *   *

The difference between the approach to Insight meditation and meditating to develop calm and concentration is summarised in a set of precepts for Mahamudra given by the Indian yogi, Tilopa, from whom the Kargyu lineage developed.

These are:

No thought,

No reflection,

No analysis,

No cultivation,

No intention,

Let it settle itself.

What these precepts are pointing to is that once you have established calm and concentration, there is no longer any need to focus on the exercises which were used to develop it. In fact, if the mind keeps returning to these exercises, they can become counter-productive.

As the meditation turns to insight the focus shifts from the meditation object itself to the process of being aware of the object. This is why meditating on space is such a good way to develop insight, for it can very easily shift to meditating on awareness. At the moment of insight there is an experience called "the turning of the mind in the seat of consciousness", and this describes the feeling of what happens when the meditation focus shifts from whatever object was used to develop the calm and concentration, to the mind itself.

In other words, for a brief moment, the mind turns to become aware of itself. This is why these precepts say to let the mind settle itself, because this is the best way to bring the process of awareness, or the mind itself, into the meditation.

*   *   *

The cultivation of mental tranquillity can be done concurrently with the foundation practices, and established through daily practice during the normal routines of our lives. Penetrative insight is usually done under retreat conditions. In the beginning, it is best to keep the periods set aside for full-time meditation work under retreat conditions reasonably short.

Starting with three days or so and then moving to one or two weeks is a good time span, for then it will always be possible to complete what was started. This is essential in developing confidence. As we are able to sustain full-time meditation work, the practice of insight will become effortless and the time in retreat can be extended to a month or more.

When calm is developed in everyday life in a relaxed manner, then the periods set aside for full-time work are not wasted and can be used efficiently and effectively.

Again, all of this work is adapted to the individual. There is certainly no need to try to undertake systematically all that has been laid out. Different aspects of the work and different ways of approaching it suit different types of people, and this is arranged in dialogue with a teacher.

Meditations for developing penetrative insight

The instructions for preparing yourself for meditating and sitting were outlined in chapter 3. There are two slight variations for Insight meditation. After you have established a calm, balanced state, you can sharpen your attention by raising the level of your eyes so that you are looking very slightly upward, just above the horizontal. Also, you can raise the tip of your tongue so that it is placed behind your top teeth.

Breathing

Breathing meditation is one of the best ways to develop Insight meditation.

Following the spontaneous movement of your breath, either watching or feeling it at the nostrils, chest or in the abdomen, is a way of bringing both the conscious and subconscious aspects of the mind together, for breathing is one of the automatic, subconscious functions of the body which can be brought to consciousness.

Meditating on space

Another form of meditation which is particularly good for developing insight meditation is taking space itself as the object of meditation.

This can be done by focusing on a visual object—one of the discs of colour for example—letting your eyes soften and half-close, and then bringing the focus of your eyes back so they are resting on the space half-way between you and the disc. Your mind will then be resting on space, which you use as the meditation object.

If you are focusing on breathing, then you can shift to meditating on space by allowing your eyes to rest on the wall in front of you and then bringing the focus of your eyes back so that they are resting on space.

Body scan

Scanning the sensations in your body is another form of meditation which can be used to develop Insight meditation.

Focusing on the sensations in your body while moving through your body from head to toe in discrete stages, keeps your body calm and your mind aware and alert.

Start at the top of the head and the forehead, noticing all the sensations there, whether pleasant, painful or even if there is no feeling in particular. Feel the tingling or pressure in the head.

Then move to the face and the lower part of the head. Soften the eyes and loosen the jaw.

Then the throat and neck, the shoulders, arms, hands and fingers.

Then move to the chest and upper back. Feel the lungs expand and contract and the movement of your ribs and diaphragm as you breathe.

Move to the abdomen and lower back and notice all the sensations there, feeling the organs moving as you breathe.

And finally notice all the sensations in the hips, legs, feet and toes. Feel or imagine the breath dropping through your body.

Once this is done your focus can then shift to resting in your head, or your abdomen, while watching or feeling the physical movement of your body breathing at that part of your body.

Truth is not an object to be grasped;
it is a state to be attained.

*The story of
the diamond*

Living the way we do is like being born with the inheritance of an extremely precious diamond and being totally unaware of its value. We ignore it while trying to gain possession of a piece of coloured glass, which to us looks magnificent and wonderful because everyone says so.

Once we have got hold of the glass we look after it carefully. We wash and polish it and display it to others, saying: "Look at what I own. It is mine. Isn't it a magnificent possession?" And eventually: "This is me." Of course everyone agrees, on the condition that you come to their house and admire their piece of coloured glass—displayed very carefully.

Some of us start to feel a little dissatisfied with our coloured glass after a while, feeling that somehow it isn't quite right—something is lacking. So we polish harder, and for some the colour starts to wear off the glass. This feels better, so we polish harder and harder, until after enormous effort all the colour is removed.

Those who achieve this are considered to be geniuses. Their glass shines and glistens and can reflect all the colours of the rainbow. They are rewarded with fame and fortune and hailed as the highest achievement of humanity.

The price, of course, is that the glass has to be kept clean and polished, so some of us find that there is still dissatisfaction, still something lacking.

We start to question and doubt and search. Is this piece of polished glass worth what everyone says it is? Could it just be an assumption without any validity?

And the doubting and questioning grow.

Everyone says: "Don't do it! You'll go blind! You'll go mad! You'll be left all alone!" But the dissatisfaction is too strong, and so we leave and face solitude in order to examine the glass and see what it is really worth.

At this stage we might meet a teacher, a friend, and ask: "What shall I do?"

The teacher says: "Give away that piece of glass you are holding."

This, of course, is terrifying. If we give up the piece of glass—the most precious object it is possible to possess—we are convinced we'll be left with nothing. And so the struggle begins in earnest. The fear arises head on, without any distraction.

The dialogue can take years—"Will I? Won't I?"—until eventually there is nothing else to do. Having reached rock bottom, we might as well admit it.

Perhaps the teacher says: "If it is easier, give it to me." So we might do so, and are horrified at the way it is treated. It isn't valued or cared for at all; it may even be casually given away to somebody else.

And so our magnificent object has gone. We are left with absolutely nothing—empty and now completely alone, with all our hopes and fears. Even these eventually start to disappear.

So we just totally give up until we become absolutely

hopeless. And we find, to our surprise, that at this stage we become completely fearless. Having stopped struggling we find that there is no abyss, nowhere to fall—we are able to rest.

Then something starts to reveal itself—without effort, without struggle—just at the moment we least expect it. Just a glimpse. We're not sure what it is, but it feels right. There's no dissatisfaction at all. The glimpses increase, until one day there is a clear view, and we see the clarity and brilliance of the original diamond.

We realise that here is our inheritance. It cost nothing. There is nothing whatsoever which had to be done to attain it or look after it—it simply is. The diamond-clear mind, free from alll concepts and mental constructions. Brilliant, open and vivid, reflecting everything yet totally ordinary.

The work we have had to do is simply in letting go of our precious possession.

We are born nameless and naked. This is our inheritance, this is our freedom. We have nothing to gain or lose—there is no "us" to look after.

This means total relief from all conflict, struggle and suffering, for there is nothing to prove or defend. No identity is separating us from others and the rest of life. There arises a state of deep, alive calm—a warm bliss, and a brilliant, radiant clarity.

To realise no-thing is worth everything.

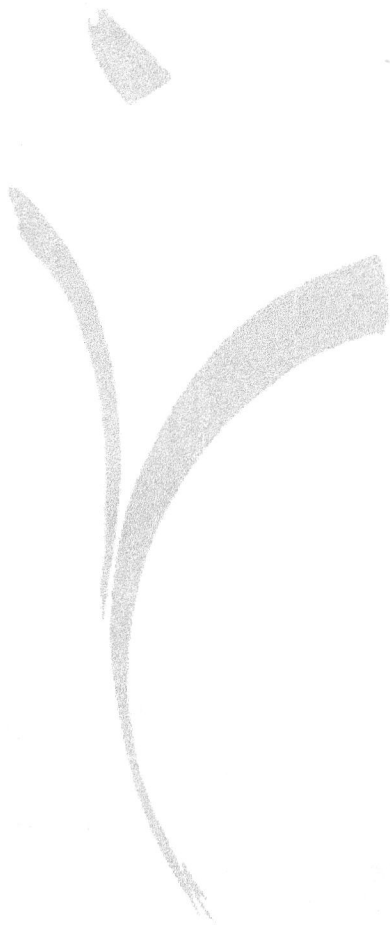

When you let go of "me" you start to be.

Freedom is not doing what we want;
it is seeing totally and clearly without preconception.

When your senses are open there are no wants,
hopes, fears or memories:
There is only seeing—no seer.
There is only hearing—no hearer.
There is only feeling—no feeler.
There is only thinking—no thinker.

CHAPTER **8** | *Integration, a life of love—going beyond wanting and fear*

After every meditation high—bliss, ecstasy and direct insight—there is a low, as the experience comes down to earth and enters daily life. The work of integration is the conscious acceptance of this; of bringing the extraordinary clarity of meditation into the ordinary experience of everyday life so that calm, clear awareness is ongoing.

There is a vast difference between simply knowing something—being able to talk about it, discuss it and explain it—and fully integrating it into our emotions and bodies so that it becomes second nature; a living experience. This means going beyond the knowledge of something, going beyond the direct experience of it, going beyond insight, and going beyond having to explain. It becomes such a natural part of our lives that it is obvious.

After every meditation high—bliss, ecstasy and direct insight—there is a low, as the experience comes down to earth and enters daily life. The work of integration is the conscious acceptance of this; of bringing the extraordinary clarity of meditation into the ordinary experience of everyday life so that calm, clear awareness is ongoing.

Calm and insight become fully realised, that is, made real, as they are lived and as the body, emotions and mind become free from states of conflict. This arises as we no longer feel that they have to be controlled, subjected to "my will"—the controller which is running the show. They are completely liberated from "my will" which becomes disengaged, even from the most subtle levels of thought and consciousness.

Liberation, therefore, is freedom from the undercurrent of craving, generated by having to want things, which normally rules our lives: wanting to control, to prove and defend our existence, to succeed or fail, to be noticed or not noticed, to be good or bad, and so on. It means going beyond the good and going beyond wisdom, for all of these are based on comparison and indicate that our minds are focused on thinking about what we are doing rather than just doing it.

Actions are either skilful, clear and fruitful, or they are unskilful, ineffective, obscured by confusion and secrecy, and eventually unfruitful. The basis of a healthy life is skilful action. Goodness can only exist in relation to evil, and so going beyond the good, going beyond love and wisdom, means not even having to think about them. There is no need to compare at all, for these qualities become a natural part of life and are totally effortless. Skilful, wise actions become truly spontaneous.

It can be seen, therefore, that spontaneity does not mean "letting it all hang out". It is the state achieved when qualities and actions have been brought to such an acute level of awareness that they are fully integrated and can be forgotten. They are an apt, direct response to what is, no matter how it might appear conventionally. Our life can then be complete and independent: not dependent on opinion or social convention.

* * *

To live in this way is to be unmoved by praise or blame, gain or loss, honour or disgrace, pleasure or pain. There is no longer any need to keep the show on the road. This is to go beyond happiness to a state of inner solitude and peace, which is the highest happiness.

Inner solitude, or inner silence, is a state of equipoise free from habitual inner dialogues. From this position it is possible to dialogue freely with everything. Nothing has to be ignored, for there is no looking for confirmation, for satisfaction, or for anything at all. Because there is no wanting, it is possible to see clearly. Inner solitude is knowing that lasting satisfaction cannot be gained from things or experiences, internal or external, for everything is insubstantial and constantly changing.

This means that there is no need to try to know about life or phenomena, for this is an attempt to grasp at them. We are able simply to allow ourselves to be one with them. This is awareness: a state of clear knowingness, completely beyond knowledge as we normally understand it.

Life cannot be grasped, it can only be lived. Therefore the only way is to enter life, trusting it, realising that we are life and that there is no "us" apart from life. In being constantly aware in our own lives, we are aware of all life. To be complete is to be not separate and, as we can never be separate from life and death, completion is the full realisation of this, in the mind, emotions and body.

*　　*　　*

The practice of meditation is based on the understanding that all action originates in the mind. Will, or volition, is the mental function of conceiving or conceptualising; of creating and shaping possibilities through decision. Once these possibilities are brought into being in the mind, they set off a train of consequences and responses. This means that what is conceived in the mind arises with certain emotions, which will induce the body to action in a particular way.

Once the mind is seen and recognised, it can be sustained in a clear, open, unconfused state, and so the actions of the body will likewise be clear, unconfused and appropriate. The ultimate solution to problems, difficulties and conflict, then, is to face them in ourselves without trying to get rid of them, for the solution is not in what should or should not be done, but in maintaining an open, healthy state of mind. This is the essence of wise action: action preceded by the understanding of wisdom.

Action can then be brought to the point where the whole idea of wisdom can be forgotten, for the mind and body become completely harmonious. Actions are then an effortless, spontaneous response to what actually is, without confusion, judgement, or concepts of right and wrong.

They are direct and immediate and have a quality of coolness to them, like a fresh breeze—neither heated nor frigid. When we are able to sense directly, with the senses, emotions and mind totally open, the whole emotional structure of habitual consciousness—the wants, hopes and fears—completely dissolves, and there is no confusion or anxiety.

*   *   *

Going beyond meditation is the point at which the distinction between daily life and formal meditation, between ourselves and what is being meditated on, dissolves, so that ordinary daily life and meditation become thoroughly mixed. What has been learned and experienced in meditation becomes an integral part of everyday life, whether in a busy, crowded city or in the open country. The highs and lows, the ecstasies and the agonies, the elations and depressions no longer have the power to overwhelm, and eventually cease to exist. They are evened out into a smooth, joyful ongoing continuum of awareness.

It is only in this state that our lives can be of use to anyone else, for then is it possible to give freely. This means that the giving is free from hope of any preconceived outcome and from looking for anything in return. As long as we are incomplete, split, there is always a level of seeking something from others.

True generosity, then, is beyond giving: a spontaneous, overflowing energy from which others can draw if they wish, or not if they don't. To be compassionate is to go beyond trying to help others, pitying them and so on, and simply opening to them; entering their pain and responding openly and freely. It is only when we have accepted and faced our own pain and freed ourselves from identifying with it, that we can see clearly the pain of others without projections.

The work of integration, therefore, is bringing the calm and insight of meditation into everyday life. It is done by bringing attention to the details of our lives while constantly referring to the feeling of calm, open clarity experienced in meditation. This, of course, requires a lot of patience with ourselves, for in the beginning we will see just how confused and painful many of the areas of our lives are.

We will also see clearly the areas which are healthy and functioning smoothly and well. Therefore, the practice of integration is to bring the feeling of calm, open clarity into every aspect of our lives. It is a feeling, a quality of mind—not something which can be worked out—developed in meditation, which can be totally infused into our lives.

There are practices which can be undertaken to do this formally; however, the best way is to give ourselves room—neither grabbing at and clinging to meditation nor grabbing at and clinging to everyday life—and after every session of meditation, take the feeling with us into whatever we do, no matter how clumsy the attempt might appear in the beginning. Eventually this will begin to show fruit, and the ultimate sign of completion is no sign at all, when all the confusion and unwholesome habit patterns have simply dropped away of their own accord, like dead leaves from a tree.

Integration involves study, contemplation, and the practice of meditation itself. In studying, we become aware of the experience and realisation of others, of the tradition of philosophy and psychology, both Eastern and Western, and of how these experiences have been formulated. From this we learn to formulate question.

In contemplation—that is, continuous reflection on the question—we learn to make it our own and bring it into our lives. In the practice of meditation, the question is brought to direct experience. This experience is then integrated into our lives.

*   *   *

Meditation is the work of love, of recognising that love is not something that just happens, but which requires discipline and understanding to be experienced and sustained. Wanting to be loved is one of the major causes of emotional conflict, for it is impossible to love or be loved without first learning to love ourselves.

This does not mean indulging in narcissism, but having true feeling for, deep understanding of, and respect for our lives. Wanting to be loved or understood is only a form of self-pity and is impossible to satisfy, for it is only possible to understand ourselves.

To love is to live; to go beyond the questions of love and hate, hope and fear, power and impotence, good and evil; to go beyond wanting to love and wanting to be loved; and opening to life. This means totally opening to desire and, through accepting it, realising that there is no-one to love or be loved.

We understand that the wanting can only be maintained by screening our perceptions and creating a fiction of an "us" which is excluded and protected from "them" and from the environment. The "us" then wants to be included. When there is no split between ourselves, others and the rest of life, wholeness and fulfilment are realised.

In order to do this, it is necessary to give up believing our own publicity, the image we have of ourselves, for it can only ever be the memory of past experience and therefore has nothing to do with what we are, what we are doing, and what actually is. This is the meaning of inner solitude: to cease dialoguing with our image of the past and to see life as it is.

It entails living our way into understanding and not trying to become something, which is just another image. Therefore, when a good belly laugh comes along, the best thing to do is to enjoy it and watch closely what is happening.

Going beyond conflict, beyond opposites and comparisons, beyond suffering, beyond life and death, is to rest in deep peace and warmth; the clear, open, luminous space of the core of our being.

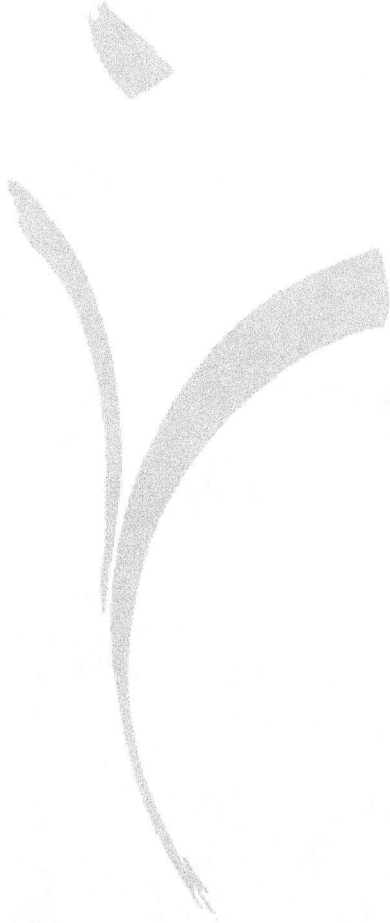

Liberation doesn't mean licence to do what we want,

it means freedom from having to want.

Everyone seeks warmth and tenderness. We feel these are due to us, and without them we feel somewhat cheated.

For the most part, our culture is emotionally untrained. We are encouraged not to not look too deeply, and when entering the realm of the emotions we often feel obliged to leave behind intelligence, and so become the victims of whatever happens to come along. This is often seen as emotional freedom and spontaneity.

We do not recognise that if emotions are unseen, unknown and unaware, there is no possibility of understanding or communicating them, and the only possible path is that of regression. This means that our emotional range becomes more and more limited and, consequently, so does our means of expression.

In order to experience and understand the aspects of life which are tender and gentle, it is necessary to recognise that the life of the emotions, or the feelings, has its own intelligence. This is an area of infinite subtlety, capable of immense refinement.

It requires patience and acute observation to come to know the range of emotional possibilities. It requires the preparedness to be completely vulnerable and receptive. Any defence or fear hardens and renders crude our perceptions, and so makes it impossible to register and recognise any but the crudest and most primitive emotions.

*   *   *

The opening of awareness to our emotions can only begin on the basis of a sense of value. This means a sense of the value of our own lives and of all life in general. It arises through observing our bodies very closely—their structures and functions—in such a way that the movement of the energies through our bodies can be sensed and felt.

Our observation is then not detached or alienated, as can happen if it is restricted to the intellect, but involves a sense of participation. Denying the feelings causes alienation, and it is this which gives rise to the devaluation of life. To observe emotionally necessitates a feeling of involvement, for it is our feelings which are being observed, and this cannot be done if we render ourselves feelingless.

Becoming aware of the fine sensings, or feelings, within our bodies leads to a feeling of connectedness with all forms of life. An awareness of the very fragile nature of all life-forms arises—the fact that they are transient and perish quickly if the circumstances upon which they depend change. It is this fragility and the transience of life-forms which gives life its value.

In observing our own body we will become aware of its transience, its vulnerability. The boredom, cynicism and sentimentality to which many people are subject often stem from the illusion that the body is permanent—the "iron man" syndrome. It is actually extremely supple, pliable and malleable, and is in a constant state of change.

The opening to the vulnerability of our body, in the depths of our being, is the experiencing of the tenderness of life. For when we face the vulnerability and impermanence of our own body, we must admit the same for all others.

The consequence of this is the realisation that it is absolutely impossible to possess another—or anything, for that matter—for both we and they are transient. Therefore, to look to another and expect that kindness and warmth must come from them, or that in possessing and holding onto someone else we will come to experience warmth, is unfair to them and impossible to fulfil.

*   *   *

It is through opening to the depth of our own being that we can come to know kindness, warmth and gentleness. For it is through facing the vulnerability and fragility of our own bodies and life processes that we will understand and value the unique constellation of forces which makes up our own lives.

In knowing this, and feeling it, we become sensitive to the feelings of others and recognise the precious quality of life. We see that for everyone and everything their life is the most precious thing they have. A full, rich and subtle emotional communication is then possible, because instead of attempting to freeze our dialogues into the rigid mould of possession, we are open to the infinite and constantly changing play of emotions within them.

As this constant play is observed, and the subtlety of which it is capable is seen, the common thread running through the variations will be discerned. This is the quality of watchfulness, of mindfulness, which brings our feelings to awareness.

It has the characteristics of coolness and evenness and can be seen as the centre around which all emotions play. As our focus moves to this quality, it will be seen that this in itself is not an emotion, but a quality of mind—a clarity. It is this which gives intelligence to feelings because from this comes the ability to discern and to distinguish.

Although the mind, in ordinary usage, is commonly associated with the brain, this particular quality of clarity is also associated with the heart region of the body. It is very fine and subtle, but once perceived and recognised, has an enormous effect on our emotions and feelings.

We are then capable of watching, learning, comparing, and sifting healthy emotions from unhealthy ones—of not being caught, trapped or manipulated into emotional dead-ends.

This is the discovery of the intelligence of the heart—a cool, clear, spacious quality of mind. This is kindness, and it gives rise to gentleness and warmth in our relationships. From this heart-space we are not acting blindly or from a position of ignorance or defence. It is possible to see and to feel clearly, and above all, to know and to recognise what we are feeling.

Relationships can then be open, free and unobstructed, as we understand clearly the play of emotions they engender, and are able to join in with what is actually taking place. This is the essence of kindness, and from this stems tenderness, warmth and gentleness.

Love is the willingness to be vulnerable.

Here we are, hurtling through space on this planet,
and yet we spend the short time we are here seeking
recognition. From whom?

To open to love is to let go of fear.

About the author

Graham Williams was born in Adelaide, Australia. He originally trained as a concert pianist, scholar and teacher, and graduated from the University of Adelaide with a Ph.D. and a Graduate Dip.Ed. He then studied in Paris for three years, and while working there realised that music was one of the few living traditions of meditation in the West. This led him to ten years' training in both the Burmese and Tibetan meditation traditions, and becoming fully ordained as a Lama by His Holiness the 16th Karmapa. During this time he spent three years in retreat and since then has spent another three years in retreat.

On returning to Adelaide, he taught at The University of Adelaide while adapting his meditation training to the Australian way of life. Interest in what he had learned and experienced led him to found The Lifeflow Meditation Centre in 1981. Graham now has nearly thirty years' experience in teaching meditation, and has trained a team of teachers who work together in the Centre. He is Director and principal teacher of the Centre, a consultant to a national company of corporate psychologists, and an Adjunct Lecturer at Flinders University. His retreats in the mallee country of South Australia, near the River Murray, have engendered a love of this timeless, peaceful, gentle yet tough land, and he has become a passionate advocate for the conservation of this unique part of Australia's heritage.

At present he is writing a series of four books based on the curriculum of the Centre.

About the Lifeflow® Meditation Centre

The Lifeflow Meditation Centre is a wholly Australian, not for profit, educational organisation founded in 1981. The Centre teaches meditation in a way that is student focused, simple and straightforward while retaining the depth of the tradition. The Lifeflow meditation technique is extremely practical, free from belief and jargon, and is easily accessible so that it can be readily integrated with everyday life. All the teachers have at least ten years of training and experience, teach from their own experience, give personal guidance, and can answer simply and directly any questions students may have. The basic courses are extremely popular, with many referrals given by doctors and psychologists.

Retreats

The Centre has two retreat properties.

Tara Hills Retreat Centre, our principal retreat centre, is set amongst rolling hills, native gum trees and an abundance of bird life in the serenity and beauty of Native Valley near Nairne in the Adelaide Hills. These features combine with the purpose-built meditation buildings which offer individual rooms and communal halls. Nourishment for the mind is accompanied by freshly prepared food for the body.

Tara Hills is only 40 minutes from Adelaide and regular public retreats are run there, from weekend retreats to 10-day retreats. Retreat themes include "Balancing Life", "Transforming Emotions", "The Joy of Being", "Dreams—myth and reality", "The Dark Night of the Soul", "Health and Healing", "Developing Awareness", "Vitality", "Wisdom", "Experiencing Union", "Insight" and "The Deeper States of Meditation".

The Kurlana Sanctuary in the Riverland comprises one thousand acres of natural scrub, which has been preserved for the wild life, and retreats are run there for members of the Centre. Here members can experience bush camping in the wild beauty of original mallee, the oldest living species of tree in the world, unique to Australia. On the property is an original pioneer house, which has been restored by the Centre and provides the venue for classes and meals.

Courses

At The Lifeflow Meditation Centre's city studio, public meditation courses are run from Monday to Friday. There are four levels from Level 1, which comprises one class per week over 7 weeks, to the advanced course. The classes are held in a spacious, well-lit room and there is ample parking available.

The Lifeflow Level 1 course provides all the experience and information needed to learn how to meditate. It covers all the different forms of meditation so that everyone can find the type of meditation which suits them. Each class takes a different topic which explains the theory behind meditation, so not only do you learn how to meditate but you also know what you are doing and why. The classes explain:

• what meditation actually is

• the different categories of meditation

• the deeper levels you experience

• how to develop awareness through meditation and use this in everyday life

• how to turn daily activities into short meditations

• how to improve concentration

• how to manage strong emotions

• how meditation relates to health, and

• how meditation can be used to open the inner life.

The Level 2 course builds on the knowledge and experience gained in the Level 1 course and spends three terms, each of 7 weeks, taking a particular topic and developing it in detail. Each term is a self-contained module so you can do just one to suit yourself or follow through the three modules of this level. The modules explore the topics of mindfulness, developing meditative concentration and balancing life. As with the Level 1 course there is plenty of time set aside for practice.

In Level 3 practice and theory are linked as in Levels 1 and 2 so that you gain the knowledge and understanding of the experiences that unfold as you build your meditation practice. Everything taught at the Lifeflow Centre is based on the direct experience of meditation, so is readily accessible and immediately applicable to your life. The classes involve active discussion and practice and each term is a self-contained module. This Level spans 8 modules over two years and covers the four streams of the meditation tradition: Calm and Concentration, Insight, Tantra and Ethics.

The advanced classes of Level 4 explore in detail the advanced levels of philosophy and psychology of the meditation tradition in a totally practical, straightforward and simple way. The knowledge you gain is integrated with our own philosophical and psychological tradition as there are many aspects which are complementary. As always, both theory and practice are linked to the realities of everyday life. This course is intended for students who have a well-established personal meditation practice and spans 8 modules over two years, covering the four streams of the meditation tradition.

The Lifeflow Meditation Centre also offers:

• retreats and workshops at Tara Hills Retreat Centre

• customised meditation training courses, either at our studio or at workplaces

• corporate programs

• courses and sessions for schools

• personal consultations to guide your meditation practice

• teacher training programs

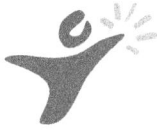

the **Life**flow
meditation centre

The Lifeflow Meditation Centre
W www.lifeflow.com.au
E info@lifeflow.com.au
P (61) 08 8379 9001

CDs and Books

Meditation CD
Graham Williams, *Experience Yourself*,
four guided meditations, Lifeflow, 2002.

Books
Eric Harrison, *The Five Minute Meditator*,
Perth Meditation Centre, Australia, 2005.
Graham Williams, *Insight and Love*,
Lifeflow Publications, Australia, 2007.

Music CDs
Reflections in Water, Piano music of Debussy,
Chopin and Liszt, played by Graham Williams.
My Heart Keeps Watch, Piano music of Olivier Messiaen,
played by Graham Williams.
Sounds of Nature, a meditation on sound.

CDs and Books can be paid for by cheque or credit
card and ordered from:

The Lifeflow Meditation Cente
Unit 8 / 259 Glen Osmond Rd
Frewville SA 5063, Australia
Ph (61) 08 8379 9001
www.lifeflow.com.au

www.ingramcontent.com/pod-product-compliance
Lightning Source LLC
Chambersburg PA
CBHW060603200326
41521CB00007B/647